Common Disorders,

Natural Remedies

A Compilation Of Previously
Published Health Articles

by: Eileen Renders N. D.
The Doctor Of Naturopathy

ISBN 0-971155   1-1-9

Copyright 2001

Renders Publishing

First Edition

Publisher's Cataloging-in-Publication
(Provided by Quality Books, Inc.)

Renders, Eileen, 1939-
    Common disorders, natural remedies : a compilation of
previously published health articles / by Eileen
Renders. -- 1st ed.
    p. cm.
    Includes index.
    ISBN: 0-9711551-1-9

    1. Alternative medicine--Popular works.   I. Title.

R733.R46 2001   615.5
                                 QBI01-201209

I

Dedication

A special thanks to friends and family who have encouraged and supported the effort and determination required to document the research, and complete the editing and producing of this book.

To Johnny my brother for his respect and belief in my dedication to this work, I will always be grateful! And for the continuing support of my husband Lucas, my daughters Linda and Eileen, my grandchildren and all of my family and friends, thank you!

May each and every one of us aspire to, and recognize the reason for our creation; To learn and to teach, for in so doing we enlarge the circle of love through sharing!

Disclaimer

The author and publisher wish to state that the educational information contained herein are in no way intended as a substitute for good medical advice, diagnosis or treatment. The Nutritional (and herbal) information and suggestions are offered only as part of Integrative Services with your physician's review and approval. While most of the recommendations contained herein are non-toxic when used according to recommended doses, occasionally they may be contraindicated in conjunction with your Medical doctor's prescribed drug therapies.

Patients experiencing strong side-effects to traditional treatment (prescribed medications) should talk to their doctor, we strongly advise against any "Self-treatment" plan.

Contents

The Circulatory, Digestive, Endocrine, Lymphatic, Nervous, Reproductive, Respiratory and the Skeletal systems may be found in part, on various pages throughout this book, but only with regard to their association and influence upon various common disorders.

INTRODUCTION

Herbs

While most Countries have long utilized Herbal Medicine as their primary medicine, the United States has been reluctant to review the possible benefits of this therapy, remaining steadfast to "traditional medicine", or Western intelligence. However, the fact remains that a great number of medicines being prescribed today owe their creation to various isolation and extractions from many types of plant species. Salicin which is the active ingredient utilized in Aspirin is derived from White Willow bark, and Digitalis often used in the treatment of heart disease is derived from the plant known as Foxglove. Taxol (paclitaxel) is a substance derived from the Pacific yew tree, and is now being used with some success in the treatment of certain types of cancers, such as; Breast, lung and ovarian cancers. And the list goes on and on.

Many Herbalists and Botanists have been writing books on the medicinal properties of herbs and plants for at least 100 years. But, the British Pharmacopeia, the Japanese Pharmacopeia and the

European Pharmacopeia have been analyzing, reviewing and documenting the hundreds of chemical constituents found in these herbs for more than 100 years. It is because of their dedication and diligent effort that the medical world is now able to reap the benefit of their effort through the rapid advancement of drug formulations brought forth into the new millennium, through the utilization of many of these herbs. Yet the first book ever written which repeatedly refers to, and which seems to suggest or confirm the healing properties contained in these herbs and plants is the Bible!

Regardless of which version of the Bible one reads, The New Testament, or The Old, these plants, flowers, and berries are mentioned over, and over again. Socrates is one of the first known Healers who implored the medicinal benefits of herbs, and his claims have been documented, and literally passed down to us over the centuries. Today however, we have world class Laboratories with Scientists and Biochemists who are finally able to document the properties which these herbs often contain, including a percentage of content.

Many of the herbs often contain such constituents as;   Tannins, alkaloids, essential oils, flavonoids, vitamins, minerals, chlorophyll, starch, mucilage, volatile oils, terpenoids, fats, sugars, resins, Amino acids, bitter principles, and saponins to name a few.

One of the first questions an individual might ask regarding herbs and their chemical constituents might be how these chemical properties differ in structure from traditional prescriptions. In order to effectively respond to such a question however, one must first be required to understand the basic philosophies and beliefs which have interested and subsequently led to the birth of Herbalists and Natural Healers since the beginning of time. One very basic philosophy is; "When one is in harmony with God and Nature, one is best able to avoid dis-ease." For those who do not believe in God, perhaps they might consider replacing Him with whatever Superior force one might believe in, but as for me, I cannot replace God in my life.

A second sensible question one might ask regarding those beliefs which are most common among Herbalists might be this one; "How does being in harmony with God and Nature help to keep us well?" The reply to that particular question is simple; "Every vitamin, mineral, or nutrient found in nature is similar in its structure, and compatible with every vitamin, mineral or nutrient found in man!" The reason for this similarity and compatibility between man and nature is that all living matter is considered organic, therefore they are easily metabolized by the human body, and efficiently utilized.

On the other hand, those chemical constituents which may have originated from, or been isolated from nature, yet have been taken to a Laboratory where their very chemical structure has been broken down for the purpose of "synthesizing", and patenting, now changes the molecular structure of what was once organic, and turning it into something that is inorganic, and incompatible with the human body. These substances (synthetic or inorganic) are not readily metabolized, nor utilized by the human body, and can be carried off and isolated in various parts of the body. Thus, the result is what is often referred to as "Side effects" which can lead to annoying symptoms.

Examples of such incompatibilities can be noted when one is taking an iron supplement which may not be easily tolerated by the body, or is not accompanied by sufficient amounts of Vitamin-C or Folic Acid, the Iron may then not be fully utilized by the body, and therefore, not provide the intended benefit. Other antagonists that can run interference could be Tannic Acid. Coffee or Tea contain a fair share of Tannic Acid, so when excess consumption of Coffee or Tea is consumed, Tannic Acid can prevent Iron from being fully utilized, regardless of how much Iron is being ingested! Other examples are readily available; An individual taking a synthetic type of Calcium for the treatment of Osteoporosis might find that a deficiency of Magnesium or Vitamin-C will interfere with the absorption of Calcium, and the Calcium being ingested could become isolated, leading to a condition known as "Calcification." Calcifications have been known to transform themselves into tumors. Tumors can in turn, become cancerous!

Another potential problem with isolating, extracting and synthesizing various chemical constituents from herbs is the potential risk of losing the effectiveness of a specific constituent's benefit, and this is often believed by Herbalists and Nutritionists to occur, when these compounds are removed from it's various other natural constituents as originally contained in, or found in nature. In other words, many Herbalists believe that by extracting or isolating a specific compound from an herb for synthesizing, one is reducing the potential of its effectiveness, as these compounds are often more effective when used in their original form, the whole herb!

"Is an herb safer for use than a prescribed drug?" The answer depends upon how it is being used. In other words, safety and effectiveness clearly depends upon the knowledge and experience of the individual making the recommendations. That is why it is strongly suggested that a practitioner who is qualified to make such recommendations be consulted, prior to any administering of such herbs. We are not all created equal when it comes to our DNA patterns, nor are any of us exactly alike with our set of illnesses, weaknesses, age, weight, or severity of specific disorders. Often, we may already be following a specific therapy, and are therefore, being administered either one or several types of medication. The bottom line is that there are considerations, and contraindications which must be addressed, all of which often precludes the idea of "Self-Treatment."

Other issues that are required when purchasing herbs are subject to the same concerns one would have when purchasing food; Purity and potency of content. While there are many Manufacturers today with Laboratories, including Chemists equal to those that we have often relied upon previously to fill drug prescriptions manufactured from huge Corporations such as Merck, Sharp and etc., so too are there now many comparable Laboratories with Biochemists who supervise the manufacture of various specific herbs.

However, we must acknowledge the fact that this is a booming industry, and there will always be those Manufacturers who are attempting to find their niche, but who have not necessarily earned their respected place as a Manufacturer who maintains the highest standards with regard to purity, and potency. This issue leads us to the next issue which is "Standardization", including what this means to you the consumer. Standardization refers to the Manufacturer's guarantee of a minimum percent of potency of the compound's "active ingredient" and will be noted on the compound's Ingredient Label. Curcumin for example is the "active ingredient" found in Tumeric. Another caution when purchasing herbs or nutrients is to look for an "Expiration date" on the bottle.

The JAMA (Journal of American Medicine Association) reported in their Nov. 1998 issue that "No longer can we look at many of these Alternative Health practitioners as Complimentary or Integrative practitioners." They went on to say that these practitioners who have studied and earned their degree, or designation (such as Nutritionist) are not only beneficial to many patients, but deserve their place in today's world as Health Care Providers.

In one study, participants were asked several questions regarding whether or not, they visited a "Holistic practitioner", or "Herbalist", and if so, how often. Included in this study were specific questions meant to target "which" type of practitioners were being visited. It appeared to confirm in the end that while most of the candidates questioned, did not have Health Insurance coverage to reimburse these individuals for their visits to such Specialists, they were willing to pay out-of-pocket costs, and did so at least three times a year.

Finally, when all participants questionnaires had been reviewed, the most visited type of practitioners were two; *Herbalists and Nutritionists!* Personally, that helped to confirm that I had indeed made the right choices earlier on in my professional career. For others, it certainly did signify where Health Care was going as the year 2000 rolled around. Many Health Care Plan Providers are now taking a closer look at what this message is relaying, and moving slowly in a positive direction toward change.

As an N. D. (Doctor of Naturopathy), and founder of RENDERS WELLNESS in Atlantic county, N. J., we have been providing Health education through Nutritional Consultations since 1995, including newspaper health articles, Lectures, Classes, and books; Food Additives, Nutrients And Supplements A To Z", The Holistic Cookbook, and more to come.

In this book, it is the author's goal to bring to the public's attention the real reason "why" so many individuals seek out practitioners who provide Consultations and non-toxic recommendations. Through research, study and practical In the-Field experience, the author will provide owners of this guide to wellness, her first hand recommendations for the management of many common, and chronic disorders of the era which prevail today. Readers will also be enlightened regarding "The Causes of Disease", including many recommendations for preventing such disorders when available.

If she is to be remembered for anything, the author would like it to be that people as a whole begin to understand the following statement; "All the best recommendations in the world would be of little value, unless one first begins to recognize, avoid and eliminate toxins and antagonists from one's body, beginning with the Shopping cart!"

Detoxification and Immune Enhancement work together in both disease prevention and/or disease treatment. Regardless of whether it is a return to good health we are seeking, or whether we are exerting the wisdom to protect the good health we have been gifted with, the information contained in this informational resource book will aid in the first step of any recovery plan.

While many of the recommendations contained herein are beneficial to most of its readers, it cannot replace the care given by a skilled Medical Advisor, or physician. That is because diagnosis, prognosis, stage of illness, as well as other drug therapy, including age and etc. must be reviewed and evaluated by a physician who has ALL of the relative information available to him/her, and will therefore become the best treatment provider.

Note: It is imperative that any therapeutic strategies that one adopts from within the pages of

*this book be **first** reviewed by attending physician!*
In selecting a physician, you may or may not
consider one who is in agreement with your own
personal beliefs and philosophies.

Nutrients And Concentrated Supplements

While much attention has been given to herbs
in the first few pages of the Introduction, in this
section we will turn our attention toward essential
nutrients and concentrated supplements. For
many years, we have heard about how deficiency
can lead to disease. The first indication may well
have been in the 1800's when Sailors aboard Ships
for many weeks often became weakened, with
gum and teeth problems, including skin disorders.
A condition known as Rickets, and a condition
that is more than rare today. When these Sailors
returned to land, and their diets began to once
again include foods containing Vitamin-C, it was
noted that all of their conditions began to subside.
And so it was discovered how the lack of Vitamin
C (an essential nutrient) could lead to a disorder.

In the 21st Century however, we have come a
long way in that we have begun to realize the
significant connection between essential nutrients

(vitamins, minerals and etc.) and disease. Without sufficient Iron, one can soon develop an Iron deficiency, or worse yet, a condition known as pernicious anemia which can often be fatal.

A deficiency of Calcium can lead to teeth problems, and recently, we have been told that an inadequate intake of fiber can cause constipation, high cholesterol, or even contribute to the onset of Colon cancer. A lack of available B+Complex vitamins can cause poor metabolism, and/or digestion of specific food types.

A lack of the EFA (Essential Fatty Acids) can also contribute to various other conditions and/or problems.

The *Essential Fatty Acids* are an essential nutrient to the health and well being of the human body, but they are not easily manufactured by the body, and best resources for them are obtained through supplementation. Without the EFA, the hair, skin and nails will eventually begin to show signs of deterioration. The EFA stimulate the release of neurotransmitters, and are therefore, especially beneficial t children diagnosed with ADD or ADHD. The EFA help to reduce the amount of Histamine produced by the body in response to allergens. They stimulate the release of Prostaglandins, and Prostaglandins are natural antiinflammatories.

Insufficient amounts of organic Sodium and Potassium will lead to lethargy as part of these Minerals functions or responsibilities is to carry nutrients to various cells throughout the body where needed. Individuals who eat poorly may indulge in overcooked foods, and as we begin to age, this along with the fact that we produce less digestive enzymes will contribute to gassiness. But, a simple supplement of Betaine Chloride (the active ingredient that works in the digestive process) can eliminate this bloating and gassiness, a common complaint of the elderly.

We've been told that in order to ingest the recommended daily allotment of fiber, we would need to eat about 5 or 6 fresh fruits daily. That would give us about 15 to 20 grams of fiber. Do you consume 5 or 6 fresh fruits daily? Bioflavonoids have been found to strengthen the integrity of our arteries, and reduce the symptoms associated with allergies. But, how can we ingest sufficient amounts, without taking a Supplement? For sure, I simply could not! But, I do take a daily supplement of a Bioflavonoid complex.

Did you know that you could lower your cholesterol considerably, without the harmful side-effects often associated with the taking of potent, often toxic prescribed drugs? It's true, you can!

ALLERGY SEASON

It seems as though we are no sooner over the Flu and Cold Season when many of us are acutely reminded that we are right back into the beginning of another Allergy Season. Studies have found that individuals who are prone to allergies are often allergic to many substances and types of allergies. Therefore, finding out what one is allergic to is often a very long and expensive procedure. In the end, many such individuals give up before the "Testing" is complete because they are found to be allergic to so many substances while they are only "Half-Way" through the Testing procedures.

Feeling a bit overwhelmed? Do not despair! For the same recommendations made for a single allergy, is usually the same advice given to those with many allergic responses.

WHAT IT IS–Whether your symptoms involve eyes, nose or the air passages and is caused by a reaction to seasonal pollens, feathers, animal hair or dust, Hay fever is a reaction of the mucous membranes and comes on an attack. When this happens, great numbers of antibodies are stimulated into action; however this chemical reaction also produces a release of histamine. And this makes the capillaries more vulnerable to the accumulation of fluid or mucous, resulting in swelling, itching, and irritation.

Magnesium is often found to be deficient and cause which attributes to crib death. It seems that a lack of magnesium in the second and fourth month of life is possible due to a baby's rapid growth. A Magnesium deficiency also is a factor in the release of histamine. Histamine is a substance that increases the permeability of the capillaries, allowing nutrients and oxygen to leak out and collect in sites such as the lungs.

A good supply of Vitamin C is necessary as it helps to eliminate toxins which accumulate within the body.

Chamomile contains a component known as Azulene, especially the German Chamomile. Azulene has helped in the prevention of allergic seizures of guinea pigs for up to one hour after administration. Azulene might also possibly help relieve hay fever in humans.

Glucocorticoids are hormones produced from the Adrenal glands, among other hormones produced by the Adrenal's and for various functions throughout the body. While glucocorticoid effect the metabolism of glucose, they also reduce inflammation and the allergic response. In circumstances of extreme stress or stress that is ongoing over a long period of time, a condition known as "Adrenal exhaustion" has been noted. In such instances, it is reported that these individuals are deficient in those hormones which help to reduce the effects associated with allergic symptoms.

Adrenal extracts are helpful, however a word of *caution* is worth noting: Adrenal extracts which are taken with out the supervision of a professional can have associated symptoms such as: Insomnia, irritability, nervousness, et cetera. In condition such as runny sinuses, open up a capsule of pure Goldenseal and pour into the palm of your hand. Holding one nostril at a time closed, with the other nostril sniff up a good portion of the Goldenseal into the other nostril. Repeat with the other nostril and you will find relief, as the

Goldenseal will dilate the passages allowing one to breath more comfortably again.

Bee pollen (not capsulated) from a jar taken in increments of ½ to one teaspoonful at a time has been shown to be a favorable treatment for some individuals, as it reduces the amount of histamine being produced in response to the allergic stimuli. Also remember that many of the pesticides used in you gardening are derived from an extract derived from the "Ragweed", a known enemy to those prone to allergies.

Many individuals have claimed to find relief from the use of Homeopathic remedies!

It is important also to understand that your Sinus problems can easily become compounded due to an infection which often does not have symptoms such as; Fever, pain, coughing or headache.

****

Almonds ~ Diabetes

by Eileen Renders N.D.   Copyright Nov., 1999

Naturally high in vitamins A, C, E, and Selenium, they also provide chromium, copper, iron, potassium and zinc. In a report released by The National Academy of Sciences, called "Diet, Nutrition and Cancer" they spelled out that the body requires a diet containing Vitamins A, C, and E, including Selenium. While Almonds do contain some fat, the type of fat is *Monounsaturated*, and monounsaturated fats are "Good" because they lower the bad LDL cholesterol, and raise the good, or HDL cholesterol levels in the blood.

While more and more Americans are gaining weight, and considered to be "Over-weight", many experts believe that malnutrition is a contributing factor. Almonds are highly nourishing, and may even offer another benefit to the Diabetic due to the fact that they are a low carbohydrate nut in comparison to others. Too, raw almonds which are coarsely ground can be utilized in recipes for making cakes and cookies, without using refined white flour! And they are naturally sweet, often requiring little to no sugar added to a recipe. For individuals with a gluten intolerance, Almond meal may be the answer.

Almonds contain 15% fat which is broken down in this manner; 75% monounsaturated, 18% polyunsaturated, and 9% saturated. The seeds of the sweet Almond tree are closely related to those of the peach tree. Almonds provide more calcium than any other nut, including iron, riboflavin, and vitamin E. Often referred to as the King of Nuts, Almonds are also abundant in magnesium, phosphorus, potassium and protein. In fact, many renown Cancer Clinics recommend 10 raw Almonds daily to their patients due to their Laetrile content. Many experts believe Laetrile to be an effective anti-cancer compound. The Oil of Almond can be dabbed on the skin after a warm bath to help alleviate dry skin problems.

Note: Avoid the salted, highly processed type, and seek out the nutritious raw form.

Aloe vera ~ From the *Liliaceae Family*

by Eileen Renders N. D.   Copyright Oct. 1999

A plant said to be first documented as a native plant of the Tropics of Africa, where related species were used medicinally as a first aid antidote to poison arrow wounds, Yet the internal gel like substance was used by both the Greeks and the Romans to treat ulcerated male genitals. Throughout the Middle ages, Aloe was used in China similarly to how it was being used in the West.

India believes Aloe gel to be a cooling tonic. By the 16th century, Aloe had reach the West Indies where is was soon being cultivated. **Constituents;** Anthraquinone glycosides, polysaccharides, gelonins, resins, sterols and chromones. **Beneficial effects;** A purgative, heals wounds, promotes bile flow, antifungal, stops bleeding, demulcent (a demulcent soothes injured or inflamed tissue, including the mucous membranes),a sedative, and expels worms. Aloe has been used for the following disorders; *Athlete's foot, ringworm, and other skin problems resulting from various types of fungi.*

7

Directions;

Apply fresh gel directly onto irritated surfaces. It can also be used as a first aid to treat small burns, eczema, sunburn, cuts, poison ivy, and chapped skin. It is also often used in Sun screens for protection against strong UV rays. Aloe vera's reduced anthraquinone content is said to be its 'Active ingredient."

Note: Aloe's leaves are hot, moist and bitter while its gel is bitter, cool, moist and salty.

Aloe vera products of today are combined with other compounds and patented, showing promise for helping to clean up our streams.

ALTERED STATES

Visualization or Guided Imagery, Self-Hypnosis and Meditation are a few of the techniques that Scientists now believe allow us the opportunity to experience, and the ability to positively affect the communication that is being carried on between the mind's memory center and various other parts of our body, such as the Immune System

A relatively new field Researchers known as Psychoneuroimmunologists, or PSNI'S are on the cutting edge of proving such discoveries. For instance, today Scientists no longer accept the notion that the human mind and the human body are separate entities. Until now Medical Studies have only concentrated on the physical evidence of an illness, utilizing all available technologies of the modern world, including CAT Scans, laser surgery, powerful medications, etcetera.

But new research in the field of PNI has shown that the brain, endocrine system, and immune systems are interconnected through a series of neural pathways. And these pathways may form a communications network which assists the body and mind in influencing one another.

The pattern which emerges is that we have long known that the seasoned Yogi in India has proven how he can control and regulate his nervous system and metabolic rate through many years of practice in meditation. Bio-feedback provides us with a device which not only provides users with information regarding their heart rate and blood pressure but can also assist them in gaining control over the same through a determined concentrated effort.

Renders Wellness also believes that when internal energy is centered and directed in a positive way, this balance and internal harmony will not only strengthen the Immune System, but will strengthen the "Whole being."

APRIL SHOWERS BRING MAY FLOWERS

By Eileen Renders N. D.

After the long winter nights, spring's milder sunny days affect our spirits as though they were smiles from Heaven above that have been mystically injected into our bodies in a form of energy that recharges our bodies to capacity for the season at hand.

It is at this time of year that the latent farmer in all of us is fighting to emerge. Flower shows, nurseries, countryside hiking, and of course, the backyard!

Whether it's tomatoes and peppers your fingers are itching to seed into the soil, or flowers are your heart's fancy, it's time to plan our strategy. In so doing, we must not forget those determined little bugs and slugs that often cause our effort at planting to go awry.

Soon some of us will also have to think about dealing with those nasty little, blood thirsty seasonal "Greenheads", better known to some as flies. Just when we thought nothing could get in our way, or stop us from enjoying our day out doors, here they come!

Perhaps this is a good time to take advantage of an opportunity to accomplish two feats in one smoothly planned effort. Why not begin your outdoor season by planting those plants and herbs which happen to be those which repel many of the bothersome insects and bugs which we have been describing? And what's more, they will be there again for you next year, affording the same protection as the year they were first planted.

These "Natural Garden Pesticides" for the most part are non-toxic, but of course you will want to make certain that small children and animals are not given a free reign to experiment!

Catnip/Catmint   While Plant attracts bees, Scent repels rats, Plant repels flea beetles

Eucalyptus ~Flea repellant

Horehound ~ Infused leaf used as a spray can repel insects. The flowering plant attracts bees.

Pennyroyal ~ Repels fleas, while a pleasant fragrance to humans. Part of the mint family with dainty blue flowers.

Caution: Pennyroyal English is Poisonous. It has small green foliage and small lavender flowers.

Rosemary ~ Labitae-Rosmarinus officinalis "alba" grows 3 to 6 feet in height. Perennial, does best in sun and well drained soil, protect from winds and cold.

Leaf; Stimulates fat digestion, when eaten and discourages insects when laid on barbecue coals. In bath water, stimulates circulation.

Tansy Compositae Tanacetum vulgare–5 feet and hardy. Ant and mouse repellent.

Caution: Can be toxic

Rue; Repels ants.

ARTERIOSCLEROSIS AND CALCIUM

While most of us have come to learn that Calcium plays a major role in the health of the human body, and is an essential element for the building of strong bones in the young, just how much Calcium is required for adults entering into mid-life, has many Experts on opposite sides of the table. Osteoporosis was once attributed to inadequate amounts of Calcium in the diet of senior citizens, today however, we now know that Calcium is only one of a number of elements which is required, and in proper balance with other minerals and nutrients, in order to maintain healthy bones, and a healthy heart. For instance; *other minerals such as Boron, copper, and magnesium, along with the vitamins C, and D must also be in adequate supply in order to maintain a healthy skeletal structure.*

Still, how many of us are truly aware of the valuable role Calcium plays in both the Circulatory and Lymph systems within the body? Admittedly, Calcium is an essential mineral, and a deficiency of long standing can contribute toward many disorders. Disorders such as heart palpitations, insomnia, and of course, Osteoporosis.   At the same time, an over-abundance of this mineral can become a huge contributing factor in the onset of Arteriosclerosis (hardening of the arteries), as well as sclerosis of the liver, skin, or eyes. Emphasis needs to be placed on the word "balance." Many individuals today are only concerned about maintaining an adequate supply of the essential minerals, as though a deficiency in one essential mineral might be the only path toward a chronic, or serious disorder. Because each essential mineral is closely involved with other minerals for stimulating healthy internal responses, proper percentage ratios of one mineral to another, is the key for determining a healthy internal mineral environment.

Excess Calcium (and more specifically, inorganic Calcium) can create a potential problem.

Organic Calcium will eagerly attach itself to carbon, oxygen, sulfur, or any number of other organic compounds, however *inorganic* Calcium cannot be effectively utilized by the organic body in the life process of a cell, therefore it is more apt to isolate, and to form a calcification, or hardening composition.

Therefore, prior to supplementing with Calcium, turn to the help and advice of one's Health Practitioner for guidance.

Tip: Organic Calcium can be found in the dark green, leafy vegetables, and in several of the herbs. Consider a Tissue Hair Analysis as a means of determining one's Mineral balance. This Test is simple, taking small samples of scalp hair. Laboratory testing is done at a Registered Lab, and will examine for 36 essential minerals, plus six of the toxic minerals; Lead, aluminum, Mercury, and etc.

****

ARTERIOSCLEROSIS-
ATHEROSCLEROSIS

By: Eileen Renders N. D.

A condition that is recognized or diagnosed by a thickening and hardening of the walls of the arteries is referred to as "Arteriosclerosis." And this disease occurs in two forms. Hardening of the artery walls that has been caused by a gradual deposit of calcium is the first type, and it is diagnosed as such because of how it is associated with the way it impairs the flow of blood to the body's cells. The other type is a more advanced type of the two, and this type of hardening is referred to as "Arteriosclerosis." And is primarily due to a buildup of cholesterol or fatty deposits in the artery walls and greatly accelerates the degeneration of those arteries involved. Too, atherosclerosis usually affects the other blood vessels of the body as well, such as the lower extremities. Fat molecules are normally absorbed through the artery walls. When an excess or overload of fatty materials begins to resist the flow of blood, fatty streaks begin to appear on the interior of the arteries. As more and more fat is introduced, the artery walls thicken and plaques of cholesterol narrow the arteries.

Partial blockage causing a limited blood supply can result in cataracts or coldness and pain in the extremities, sometimes leading to gangrene. Lack of sufficient blood supply to the brain causes confusions, senility, and strokes. Angina attacks can happen when any restriction of blood flow is being experienced near the heart. And a clot can form anywhere in the body and work its way to the brain or the heart.

Some of the symptoms often associated with atherosclerosis might be: hypertension, cramping or paralysis of muscles, sensation of heaviness or pressure in the chest or pain which might radiate from the chest to the left arm and shoulder.

RISK FACTORS: Lack of physical activity, smoking, obesity, hypertension, stress, and a faulty diet, and possibly heredity.

It is important to understand that it is not always one's diet which causes an abnormally excessive accumulation of fat within the arteries. Studies have shown that in certain individuals the liver itself (which is where cholesterol is manufactured, as we all need a small amount of cholesterol for optimum functioning) makes far too much cholesterol, owing to the heredity factor.

The essential fatty acids along with vitamin E are necessary for the maintaining the health of the arteries, among other things. But it should be realized that through the processing and refining of certain foods, vitamin E along with the essential fatty acids are completely lost.

Those who may be facing the reality of a triple bypass surgery would be wise to make certain that they have gotten a second opinion to say the least. And they would be better able to make sound decisions in reviewing the total picture, literally! By this I mean that one should examine thoroughly the extent of one's disease process and know one's options.

In other words, those who have tiny blockages which are not near the heart might inquire as to how diet, regular exercise and oral chelation might work for them. There are also medical physicians who believe in and provide just such services. Again oral chelation might be only for those who have minor problems and will therefore be able to wait for the changes of a slow reversal to take shape through such a program. Others might find it worth their while to look into the potential of opting for chelation intravenously (it is much faster, but of course more costly). Still there will be those who should heed their medical physician's warning and undergo the triple bypass. Yet even for those, all would be in vain, were each of these survivors not to recognize the need for initiating healthier positive changes in their lives.

Note: There are various types of Calcium utilized for supplementation, but not all types are easily utilized nor metabolized by the human body. Chose a type which is compatible, Calcium citrate is said to be most compatible, but should be taken in graduated doses until maximum dose recommended by your Nutritionist has been met. This will help to avoid the potential for diarrhea.

ATHEROSCLEROSIS

by: Eileen Renders N. D.

Copyright August, 2000

A disease marked by fatty deposits within the artery walls, these fatty deposits eventually develop into a plaque which causes obstruction of blood flow.

As far back as the middle fifties, renown Nutritionist Adele Davis provided insight into this disease (backed up by Scientific research) which explains how Lecithin, a nutrient made by the body, but only when sufficient amounts of specific B-vitamins are available In the body such as B-6, Choline, and Inositol, helps to break-down cholesterol into tiny particles which are able then to pass through the body's tissues. Only when we are deficient in Lecithin does cholesterol become large, thus getting trapped in the blood and arterial walls.

Cholesterol deposits interfere with how oxygen is supplied to the brain. Lowering blood cholesterol increases the oxygen supply and speeds recovery!

Lecithin contains;   Fat, Choline, Inositol, and unsaturated fats.

*Vitamin B-6 and Magnesium assist the body in making Lecithin.

The Essential Fatty Acids (Linoleic and Linoleic) can also be supplemented through the implementation of Organic Flax Oil.

To insure sufficient amounts of Inositol, Choline and linoleic acid (essential nutrients which help to maintain optimum transport and functioning of human cells, is to supplement daily with Lecithin made only from pure Soy granules. Lecithin made from pure Soy granules is an excellent source for Inositol, Choline and Linoleic acid.

FOODS TO AVOID

Hydrogenated oils such as;   Palm kernel, Coconut, Peanut & etc. Hydrogenated oils are oils which are heated at extreme temperatures which break down the molecular structure and destroy its nutrients, turning them into potential carcinogens.

Hydrogenated oils are also capable of destroying the body's supply of essential fatty acids (the "good" fatty acids such as Linolenic and Linoleic.

Nitrates and Nitrites: Such as are found in Hot dogs, sausages, luncheon meats, smoked meats and etc. Nitrates and Nitrites form a chemical reaction within the intestines known as "Nitrosamines", potentially dangerous carcinogens.

Limit amount of meats eaten weekly such as; Lamb, pork and beef, as they contain a fair amount of saturated fat, fats which have the potential of contributing to high blood cholesterol levels.

****

BLACK COHOSH (herb)

By; Eileen Renders N. D. Copyright 1997

Many people today are taking a longer look at herbs for the relief of annoying symptoms, and for other beneficial effects. And while herbs have always been a part of my recommendations, some are nonetheless, capable of creating an internal toxicity when used inappropriately in the hands of one who is experienced, or when used to excess. Others may also be inadvisable when used in conjunction with other medications.

Contraindications for a particular herb that is utilized for its reputed effects can create an extreme potency when combined with certain prescribed drugs. In other words, implementing a natural diuretic such as *Cornsilk,* while implementing a regular routine of exercise (along with other specific nutrients), while at the same time one is taking a medication to manage one's "Borderline" blood pressure (a blood pressure reading of 145/90) could cause the blood pressure to suddenly take a 180 degree turn and drop below what is considered normal i.e., 120/80.

In my practice, people often tell of taking one or another of the "Herbs" because *They heard it was good.* Yet while they may have some accurate information regarding a particular herb they have begun to use in a self-treatment plan, often they *do not* have all of the information necessary to successfully carry out a therapeutic protocol. For instance, without full knowledge on the contraindications often associated with the herbs, the chances of making an error in dosage or duration are increased. ***Black Cohosh*** may be one such herb that has recently been over-ingested, without proper knowledge. Its chemical constituents include alkaloids, tannins terpenoids, and several other constituents. Black cohosh is said to possess antirheumatic, antitussive (a drug that suppresses coughing), sedative, and emmenagogue (an agent that stimulates menstruation properties.) Today, it is widely used for everything from irregular menstruation to PMS (Premenstrual Syndrome). Yet, Black Cohosh carries contra-indicators, warnings, and side-effects which are often unknown to the buyer.

Contra-Indications: This herb should not be used by pregnant of lactating mothers. Studies show that black cohosh binds to uterine estrogen receptors. An over-dose may cause premature births. ***Warnings***: It has been recommended that black cohosh should only be used in therapeutic doses and that high doses are potentially dangerous. ***Side-effects and toxicity:*** Overdoes may produce symptoms of nausea, vomiting, dizziness, visual and nervous disturbances, together with reduced pulse rate and increased perspiration. ***Acetin*** (one of several terpenoids contained in black cohosh) is one of the "ctive" ingredients in black cohosh, and one which has not yet been fully studied.

Recommendations: Seek the advice and supervision of a professional.

Black cohosh *Cimicifuga racemosa*

Chaste-tree berry *Vitex-agnus-castus **And***

***PMS** ~ Pre-Menstrual Syndrome*

by Eileen Renders N.D.

Copyright Nov. 1999

PMS has various symptoms such as mood swings, irritability, nervousness and etc., and is often associated with stress (physiological and/or emotional) and is experienced at various levels or degrees of seriousness.

Black Cohosh is an anti-spasmodic and sedative herb which has long been used by herbalists for balancing the nervous system, and as a tonic. It can be taken in combination with such herbs as Lemon balm, Passionflower, and/or Valerian root for a relaxing effect.

Recommendations: A standardized extract of 200 Milligrams of 2.5% Triterpene Glycosides is best.

Two capsules taken once daily (A.M. & P.M.)

Beginning at onset of monthly menses for two weeks, followed by two capsules twice daily for the remainder of the month. Repeat for three months, cease for one month, and then begin again.

Chaste-tree berry herb, along with a regular routine of exercise, and good nutrition can help to alleviate annoying symptoms associated with PMS and often caused by hormonal imbalances. Abundant in flavonoids, monoterpenoids and steroids among other constituents, Chaste-tree berry has long been utilized by herbalists for enlarging the mammary gland , and to increase lactation due to its effect upon the pituitary gland.

Recommendations: An extract of 150 Milligrams containing 0.5% Agnuside in capsule form, a dose of 450 Milligrams taken once daily for three weeks, and then discontinued for the last week of the month.

Caution: *Pregnant, or Lactating women should avoid taking herbs, without physician's knowledge.   Others should seek professional Consultation in order that all medical diagnosis be reviewed, including contra-indications regarding any current medications.*

As always, individuals taking Insulin, or ACE inhibitors should seek medical advice!

****

Blackberry *(Rubus villosus)*
by: Eileen Renders N. D.
Copyright Sept., 2000

Natural Order goes by the name of Rosaceae, and includes more than 1,000 species. Found most abundantly at one time in Australia, it grows in many parts of the world. This plant with its succulent berries has been mentioned and utilized as far back as when the ancient Greeks used blackberry as a treatment for gout. To begin to attempt to understand the graces bestowed from the blackberry, one must first recognize a few common biochemistry facts. For example;   Citrus fruits contain acid (lemons, limes, grapefruits and etc.). In looking at 21 parts of citric acid, aside from its water content, about seven atoms of oxygen is available from same. But, in apples, blackberries, raspberries and etc., there are other acids present, including Malic acid, which provides 1/3 oxygen. In elderberries, cherries, plums and prunes and etc., we find yet another acid known as tartaric acid, an acid which provides 6 from 16 parts of available oxygen, including potassium, magnesium, iron and potassium.

Tannic acid is found in astringent herbs (such as berries, leaves, nuts, barks and roots), however tannic acid carries a bit less oxygen than previous mentioned herbs. Tannic acid is eventually converted into gallic acid. These acids are known for their ability to tone and eliminate excess mucous, and also lends itself well (understandably) as a preservative.

Yet none can be compared (to quote Dr. Shook) with the blackberry because of its generous oxygen content, as well as its iron content which wins hands done for its curative powers for building up the blood, carrying oxygen to every human cell, and the cleaning up of waste matter and debris as it renews life's energy to every living cell.

Blackberry ~ The berries eaten fresh contain Citrate, malate, and tartrate of iron, potassium, calcium, sugar, gum and coloring matter. Medicinally they have been utilized in a *Cordial,* as a tonic, astringent, oxygen carrier, blood maker, cardiac tonic, solvent of calcarious deposits, antiseptic and as an anti-arthritic.

Notes;   The leaves are less potent and therefore, often used for children. One ounce of blackberry leaves to I pint of boiling water, steep for 10 minutes. Strain and add a bit of honey. It can be given in doses of One tablespoonful to children with diarrhea.

****

CALCIUM AND DEPRESSION

A recent report from clinical psychologist Dr. Richard Malter who is the Director of the Malter Institute for Natural Development in Illinois, states that serious psychological problems can result from extended use of calcium supplements. Other adverse conditions associated with calcium supplementation might include fatigue, exhaustion, depression, anxiety, panic attacks, headaches, paranoid feelings, loss of memory and concentration, headaches and insomnia.

An example is a patient who had just celebrated her fortieth birthday and had read in her local newspaper about the dangers of osteoporosis attacking women her age. Consequently she began to self-medicate with Calcium supplements. Soon thereafter she became depressed. Months later she was engulfed in waves of depression, coupled with fits of anger and crying spells for no apparent reason, and even became suicidal. After attending a lecture by the doctor, she put two and two together and realized that her problem began after starting the calcium supplements. She consulted with Dr. Malter, who advised that she obtain a TMA (Tissue Hair Analysis). In the meantime he suggested that she discontinue the calcium supplementation. Within a very short time the anxiety attacks disappeared, the depression lifted and her mental health returned. It should be noted that the TMA confirmed that this patient should not have taking calcium supplements at that time.

Another example is a doctor who was treating a woman for depression for four years, without a positive response. After reading the above published article, he decided to physically visit the laboratory where the Tissue Hair Analysis testing was being conducted by Dr. Malter. Relating his treatment of the above referenced woman for four years without noting any progress, it was decided that a TMA be completed on that woman. And after reading the results of the TMA (Tissue Mineral Analysis) and speaking with the woman they learned that she too had been taking calcium supplementation for four years. TREATMENT: Soon after ceasing calcium supplementation, she too was returned to a healthier psychological state. These women were what is known as "Slow

Metabolic Types" states Dr. Malter. Slow metabolizers are more likely than fast metabolizers to develop psychological problems when they take calcium supplements to correct a calcium disorder. A Slow Metabolizer Type individual requires a much different approach to correction of calcium disorders.

Other factors associated with too much tissue calcium include: Susceptibility to viral infections. Studies have shown that when calcium is added to tissues containing dormant viruses, the virus will become more active and proliferate readily. Blood calcium circulating in the blood should not be confused with tissue calcium. The body's tissue calcium balance is not always associated with abnormalities in the serum calcium. Hypocalcaemia is a relatively rare clinical problem. It occurs when the total serum calcium falls below 7 milligrams percent. Chronic renal failure, intestinal malabsorption problems, and an inactive parathyroid gland are usually associated with this problem. When circulating calcium falls below a certain threshold, hyper irritability can ensue. Another danger is "tetany," a condition that causes periodic and painful muscular cramps and even seizures. If the condition becomes severe, the sufferer can die due to respiratory failure.

Hypercalcemia is a condition defined as having a serum calcium above 10.5 milligrams percent. However, symptoms of the condition may not appear until the serum calcium reaches 12 milligrams. Paget's and Addison's disease are associated with hypocalcaemia as well as the use of diuretic medications.

VITAMIN-MINERAL SYNERGISTS:

By: Eileen Renders N. D.

Synergistic to calcium (absorption of calcium) is Vitamin D, Vitamin C, Vitamin E, and Vitamin A, along with other minerals.

In the case of Hypercalcemia, another protocol would be recommended in order to excrete excess calcium, along with ceasing supplementation of same.

FINAL NOTE: In serious conditions, such as those noted above, do not attempt to self-medicate and NEVER fall victim to the theory or practice that includes More is Better!

■■■

CANCER/EXERCISE

The University of California at Berkeley recently provided their findings and opinions regarding cancer and how to best prevent the same. In 1996, I provided an informal health lecture regarding the very same topic to a group of cancer survivors, but was very discouraged to realize that this particular group was not interested in hearing anything which might indicate a change of lifestyle was necessary. Nor were they ready to make an concessions regarding limiting the amount of those "Favorite" foods they had become accustomed to, let alone put forth any real effort into the theory regarding how exercise could strengthen their bodies attack against free radicals activity. In fact, it is my opinion that these individuals were really looking for a "Quick-fix magic pill" which would guarantee a long and healthy life. Needless to say, I was aghast! For were it me, I would have been willing to go to any lengths to protect and strengthen my body and not only lengthen my life but enhance the quality of it.

Today, however, many universities such as the University of California at Berkeley, which I am quoting here, are advocating just such changes in everyone's lifestyle. Exercise reduces one's chances of developing heart disease, diabetes, stroke, and osteoporosis. It helps to ward off Osteoarthritis and the mental decline that can develop in middle age. But it might possibly even be a good defense against colon cancer. Exercise helps in maintaining one's idea weight, boosts the metabolism, and strengthens the immune system. It can prevent obesity and exercisers have a lower risk of dying prematurely from chronic diseases than so sedentary people.

Exercise stimulates the internal organs into performing optimally, thereby preventing fluid accumulation and/or constipation. It enhances the circulation which in turn increases the utilization of oxygen. All of which increases one's available energy. It stimulates the production of hormones which effect one's mood, and can overcome some forms of mild depression caused by hormonal imbalances. Need I say more?

Yet often the first reply to such information are all of those excuses of why one simply cannot exercise: I'm too tired; I have a bad back; I have bad feet; I have a weak heart; I don't have time; I don't have enough energy and on and on and on. Certainly one with diabetes or a bad heart should surely consult with one's medical physician before instituting an exercise program. But often walking or water exercises are encouraged even for those with such complaints. Essentially, all one needs for walking is a good pair of shoes.

See your medical physician and stop procrastinating and get started! See the fall leaves this year on your bike.

CANCER RISK FACTORS

Second only to cardiovascular disease, cancer is responsible for over 400,000 deaths year. When healthy body cells suddenly enlarge and divide, they become incapable of providing any usefulness or protection to the body. This radical change is known as *carcinogenesis*. Cancerous cells have a unique ability to grow rapidly, without order or predictability. Some cancers will remain in their primary site of origination, and others will *metastasis* (randomly) move throughout the body, establishing secondary sites). Some forms of cancer will provide rapidly, taking over a specific organ of the body rendering it inoperable. Others may grow very slowly, avoiding detection for many months, or years.

While there are several research theories regarding *how* cells are injured, it is agreed by most that many *carcinogens* (cell damaging-cancer causing agents) are associated with the onset of cancer. Therefore, avoidance of these carcinogens is one of the exert in the prevention of cancer. Managing stress and exercising can help to protect the immune system, as will institution of

40

healthier nutritional choices. Avoidance of tobacco smoke (which is thought to be the leading cause of lung cancer) is another way in which we can protect ourselves from cancer. **What are some of these carcinogens, and where are they commonly found?** They can be found in many processed foods in the form of *additives*. They are often an ingredient found in many cleaning agents, insect repellants sued for growing produce, or nitrates found in many luncheon meats, or smokes meats such as bacon. Here is a partial list of many *suspected carcinogens*: Artificial sweeteners, asbestos, aspartame, caffeine, conjugated equine estrogen, decaffeinated coffee, drinking water, fat, hair dye, herbicides, mouthwash, ultraviolet radiation, and vinyl chloride.

Choose fresh fruits and/or vegetables whenever possible, and rinse your vegetables and fruits well. Peel off the outer leaves of lettuce, cabbage, et cetera before eating. Follow a low-fat diet (avoiding an over abundance of deep fried foods), trim the fat from your red meat, and when possible choose quality cuts of meat (sacrifice quantity for quality). Consume adequate fiber, and include a daily antioxidant along with your multi-vitamin.

CAUSES OF DISEASE

By: Eileen Renders N. D.

In this particular article, we shall explore some of the "Causes of disease@ and attempt to explain exactly how each of us might be able to affect positive changes in our health. While the many types of disease are too numerous to list, their originations may not be so difficult to pinpoint. Andy they are:

Congenital deformity ~ (a disease or deformity one has been born with or inherited)

Hereditary weakness ~ A pre-existing factor, which makes one more prone to a particular disease or condition.

Organic injury ~ This might best be explained by a sudden traumatic injury or "Accident."

Cellular Contamination ~ While there are many such diseases, cancer is one that is often associated with same.

Nutritional Deficiency ~ A condition which may be transient or chronic. However, unnoticed or unchecked over a long period of time, can become acute leading to vulnerability and disease.

43

might expect to be answered correctly by all might be this one: "Which of the above circumstances might each of us most probably be able to influence or correct?"

If you answered, "Nutritional Deficiencies" you would be correct! Therefore, we would then have learned an important lesson. Recognizing and correcting nutritional deficiencies is our responsibility, for the most part. For those who are not certain about their body's needs and/or requirements and how they relate to one's daily nutritional choices, it would be wise to seek the advice of a professional.

Too, keep in mind that the RDA's recommendations are this "A Minimum Recommended Daily Requirement." All things are not equal, and each of us due to separate inherited and environmental circumstances may require more or less of a particular vitamin or mineral in order to correct a deficiency of long standing.

Make nutritional choices for your body based on what that food can do for your body, rather

than a compulsion or an addiction to a denatured
or devitalized food.

Smile And Say Cheese...Cake

By: Eileen Renders N. D. Copyright 1997

As promised in my last column, here is a cheesecake recipe which can accommodate most of us. While the cream cheese version will be richer, for those with an intolerance or on a strict low-fat diet, tofu will lend itself nicely.

FILLING

- 16 ounces of cream cheese, tofu or drained yogurt (If tofu is your choice, the silken tofu may be more desirable to the firm)
- ½ cup of fructose or Sucanat
- 2 teaspoons of lemon juice
- 3 eggs, slightly beaten or egg substitute
- 1-1/4 cups of plain yogurt or tofu
- 1 tablespoon unbleached flour or oat flour

DIRECTIONS

Combine the cream cheese, fructose and lemon juice in a processor or blender, add slightly beaten eggs and yogurt. Pour into desired crust (a graham cracker crust would enhance the flavors). Bake at 350 degrees for about 45 minutes.

- 1 cup plain drained yogurt (or vanilla yogurt) and/or ½ substitute cream cheese (low fat)
- 3 tablespoons fructose
- 2 teaspoons vanilla

DIRECTIONS

Mix together ½ cup of yogurt and ½ cup of substitute low-fat cream cheese, fructose and 2 teaspoons of vanilla, spread over top of baked cheesecake and bake an additional 15 minutes or longer. Chill before serving. Add sliced strawberries, pecans or fruit preservatives prior to serving.

■■

How To Lower Cholesterol Naturally

by Eileen Renders N.D. Copyright 1999

Latest surveys find that of the thousands upon
thousand of individuals who are prescribed a
blood lipid-lowering medication, only half are
following their Doctor's recommendations. I'm
not surprised! It seems to be one of the most over-
prescribed drugs on the market today (along with
Ritalin for ADD.) While high cholesterol is
certainly one of the risk factors associated with
heart disease, it is should not be singled out, nor
over-emphasized. In fact, there may be a
difference of "Professional opinion" regarding
what is considered high, as that number has
changed a couple of times in the last several years,
just enough to include a higher number of people
who belong in the category that should be taking a
drug. Then we are warned; "But, be careful, as
you may need to have regular Liver tests done!"
And, if you have Liver disease, are pregnant,
nursing, or have any other medical problems, tell
your Doctor about them. That message is
confusing, and maybe that is why many are not
taking their medications faithfully. Maybe, our

instinct tells us that we are not willing to trade a healthy Liver, for a "Good" cholesterol reading.

HOW TO INTERPRET YOUR CHOLESTEROL RESULTS ~ First of all, a cholesterol reading will include the following types of readings; LDL (or bad cholesterol), total cholesterol reading (highest number reported), the HDL (or good cholesterol) which effectively escorts "Out" the bad cholesterol, keeping your arteries free from plaque build-up. By the way, individuals with a predisposition to high cholesterol usually have heavy plaque build up on their teeth. There is also another reading called VLDL, however most Laboratories do not provide this reading. So here is a scenario for you to toss around, and help you understand what high cholesterol means; Suppose you have a LDL reading of 280, and an HDL reading of say 70. What you need to do is divide the 280 (considered time for medicine reading) by the HDL number, which in this scenario is 70. What you now get is a number of 4.0. Now, let's do a typical comparison; Let's say I have a fairly good LDL number of 220, but my HDL is only 35. After we have properly done our math, we come up with a ratio number of 6.3. Ratios are meant to our math, we come up with a ratio number of 6.3. Ratios are meant to determine how effectively one=s HDL (good cholesterol) is escorting out the bad cholesterol, therefore they are an index which measures one=s Risk Factor for a Stroke, or heart attack! As you can see, the individual with the higher cholesterol number is in a safer index than (hypothetically) me who had the lower LDL number, *or where do we go with that total cholesterol number?*

Well, now we need to examine whether or not, there are other risk factors involved which might add to the high cholesterol risk, in order to effectively determine how we really feel about taking our medicine.

Other Risk factors are;

1.-Obesity

2.-Sedentary Life-style

3.-Diabetes

4.-Stress

5.-Cigarette Smocking

6.- Poor nutrition

7. Deficiencies in EFA, and

Antioxidants

What else remains to be said?

Thousands of individuals believe today that "If" they have a good cholesterol reading that they are somehow protected, or will be spared from a fatal heart attack as they begin to age. Rarely however, do those individuals understand the concept of protecting the health of their arteries. Besides Atherosclerosis (vessel blockages due to cholesterol, or fibrin accumulation), there is yet another artery disease known as Arteriosclerosis which is disease of the arteries caused by loss of strength, and resilience. Arteries can rupture, or break leading to a Stroke.

Recommendations: Include a sufficient amount of EFA ~ Essential Fatty Acids into the diet (Flax oil is best), raw carrots, psyllium, Vanadyl sulfate, rice bran capsules and Red yeast rice, all found at your local Health Food Store.

Concentrated Rice Bran Capsules are non-toxic and just two capsule per day will lower your total lipid blood levels approximately 15 to 20% in as little as Five weeks. All the more reason to avoid toxic drugs which threaten to cause adverse side effects to the body's main filtering agent, the Liver! Always have a total blood lipid Test done prior to beginning on your Cholesterol lowering campaign, and again about 5 to 6 weeks after embarking on same!

Preventing Colds and Flu

by Eileen Renders N.D.   Copyright 1996

With the flu and cold season upon us, it makes good sense to turn our attention toward the immune system. What is it and how does it protect us?

The thymus, which is part of one endocrine system, plays a vital role in helping keep us well. Located just behind the breastbone, the thymus gland is responsible for the development of the immune system. It produces cells called lymphocytes. These lymphocytes are coded early on so that they will recognize invaders within the body's tissues. In adults lymph nodes, bone marrow and the spleen will contribute to protecting the immune system by producing lymphocytes.

Both the red and the white blood cells also play a vital role in helping the body to protect us from disease. While it is the red blood cells which provide the cells oxygen and assist in escorting out carbon dioxide, it is the white blood cells known as leukocytes that defend against attack. The largest of the white blood cells, called macrophages are the largest type and are capable of eating up a whole colony of bacteria.

Certain essential nutrients act to strengthen our immune resources, such as vitamin P or bioflavonoids. Brightly colored, water soluble substances, they often are available in fruits and vegetables along with vitamin C. The components of bioflavonoids are citrin, hesperidin, rutin, flavones and flavonals. Sources are available in lemons, plums, grapefruit, grapes, black currants, apricots, cherries, blackberries, buckwheat and rose hips.

Bioflavonoids are reportedly nontoxic. Besides enhancing the immune system, bioflavonoids have been used successfully in the treatment of such diseases as arthritis, rheumatic fever, gynecological problems, duodenal ulcers (with special diet), inner ear disease and rheumatoid arthritis.

Coenzyme Q-10 or Co-Q-10 is a natural concentrated supplement derived from the flavonoids and can be purchased in various strengths such as 10 to 100 milligrams.

A 60 milligram daily supplement added to one's diet during the winter season is a good way to boost the immune system and while it may not stave off a cold or the flu, it can reduce the severity and shorten the duration.

****

Diabetes/Beneficial Herbs and Nutrients

by Eileen Renders N.D.   Copyright 1999

Sugar cravings have been linked, according to many nutritional experts, to the body's attempt to restore and/or maintain adequate serotonin levels. The unsaturated fats (essential fatty acids ~ linoleic and linolenic acids) assist the body to stimulate the production and uptake of serotonin, thus leading to a clear mind, and sense of well being.

Vitamin-B6 (part of the B complex vitamin) can also assist in alleviating sugar cravings. Rather than supplementing this vitamin alone, it should be taken in combination with a B+complex vitamin in order to eliminate other B vitamin imbalances. 100 Milligrams is a suggested dose.

Chromium picolinate~ Employed by insulin, chromium assists cells to better utilize glucose, and a deficiency in this element raises the body's requirement for insulin. And since insulin contributes to the body's excretion of chromium, diabetics dependent on insulin injections often have a pronounced chromium deficiency.

Fenugreek~ *Trigonella foenum-graceum* This herb dates back as far as Hippocrates. Egyptian women regarded it as an aid in easing the pain associated with childbirth, and it was often recommended to nursing mothers to insure a healthy supply of milk. Containing mucilage, saponins, alkaloids, protein, vitamins and minerals, Western researchers have found this herb to have a "Hypoglycemic" effect. In some studies using urine samples, it was shown to cut in half existing sugar levels.

Ginseng~ Chinese pharmacology indicates that this herb has been shown in Laboratory studies (with animals) to stimulate the release of insulin from the pancreas, and can also support adrenal gland function.

Vitamin E~ This potent antioxidant assists the body in better insulin reaction, and is therefore beneficial to diabetics. Vitamin E may help in preventing cardiovascular disease, secondary to diabetes.

Zinc~ A mineral which assists in regulation of the body's energy supply, it is one of the substances which comprise what constitutes the hormone insulin.

Sugar substitute~ An herb known as Stevia for your daily cup (one) of coffee. Remember that Aspartame, and various other sugar substitutes are on the "Suspect" list of carcinogens, as is caffeine.

****

DIGESTIVE PROBLEMS ~

At some time or another, most of us have been the victim of the many symptoms often associated with Dyspepsia (indigestion) is "Impaired digestion." Such symptoms often include: bloating, flatulence, belching, burning, diarrhea, constipation or nausea. While the information offered here is not meant for a substitute for a total Medical examination (for those who suffer these symptoms regularly) in order to rule out more serious causes for these symptoms, it may be useful for those who are simply experiencing the effects of faulty life-style habits such as: decreased physical activity (as often noted in the elderly and/or debilitated), poor nutritional choices, insufficient digestive enzyme production, allergic reactions, chronic Candida, et cetera.

A few simple suggestion may be just enough to reverse this problem for many, and they are as follows:

1. Chewing food thoroughly will help to increase the amount of saliva which contains the first digestive enzyme needed in the process of

"breaking down" food molecules and this enzyme is known as amylase.

2. Eating more raw foods is helpful as this is where many of the enzymes required for the continued process of digestion can be obtained.

3. Drinking a sufficient amount of water with each meal is another way of increasing the proper metabolism (anabolism and catabolism) of each meal.

4. Often it may be simply the food itself! Some individuals are often sensitive to rich creamy sauces, or highly spiced foods. Too, it may be helpful to understand how certain food combinations are more difficult for the body to digest.

Also, over-loading the body with huge meals can be the problem. Eating smaller meals at shorter intervals may often relieve digestive problems.

5. Eating when one is in a hurry or stressed can often impair digestion causing malabsorption.

As we begin to age our bodies do not supply sufficient amounts of needed hydrochloric acid. Hydrochloric acid is the main ingredient responsible for the break-down of ingest foods,

and helps us to maintain the proper internal ph.
RECOMMENDATIONS: A half-hour before
each meal, take a couple of papaya supplements.
These are very pleasant tasting and contain one of
the digestive enzymes (papain). They can be
found at your local health food store. CAUTION:
Those who experience pain, nausea, and/or
continued and prolonged digestive problems
should visit their medical physician to undergo
diagnostic tests. *Also. Have your practitioner (or
Nutritionist) provide you with a List of Acidic,
Alkaline and Neutral foods and limit acidic types.*
NOTE: When all serious conditions have been
ruled out, one might consider a consultation to
learn more about food combining and other
helpful recommendations at Renders Wellness, or
a qualified Nutritional practitioner in your area.

EMPHYSEMA ~

Emphysema is a condition in which there is an over inflation of structures in the lungs known as *alveoli* or air sacs. This over inflation results from a breakdown of the walls of the alveoli, which causes a decrease in respiratory function (the ways the lungs work) and often breathlessness. Early symptoms of emphysema include shortness of breath and a cough. Emphysema is a widespread disease of the lungs. It is estimated that 70,000 to 100,000 Americans living today were born with a deficiency of a protein known as alpha 1-antitrypsin (AAT) which can lead to an inherited form of emphysema. Emphysema ranks ninth among chronic conditions that contribute to a person's lack of activity. Many of the people with emphysema are older men, but the condition is increasing among women.

Causes: Scientific research has shown that the lung has a remarkable balance between two classes of chemicals with opposing action. It also has a system of elastic fibers. The fibers allow the lungs to expand and contract. When the chemical balance is altered, the lungs loose their ability to balance is altered, the lungs loose their ability to protect themselves against the destruction of these elastic fibers. This is what happens in emphysema. Several reasons cause this chemical imbalance. **Smoking is responsible for 82 percent of chronic lung disease, including emphysema.** Exposure to air pollution is another suspected cause. Irritating fumes and dusts on the jobs also are thought to be a contributing factor. Still, a small number of individuals with emphysema have a rare inherited form of the diseased called *Alpha-1-antitrypsin (AAT) deficiency-related emphysema,* or early onset emphysema. This form of disease is caused by an inherited lack of the protective protein called AAT.

Note: Emphysema doesn't develop suddenly it comes on very gradually. Years of exposure to the irritation of cigarette smoke usually precede the development of emphysema. An initial symptom as usually described to the doctor is the sudden feeling of shortness of breath during activity or exercise. As the disease progresses, a brief walk can be enough to bring on difficulty in breathing. **Some people may have had chronic bronchitis before developing emphysema.**

Treatment (best treatment is prevention) and other suggestions: The single most important factor for maintaining healthy lungs is to **QUIT SMOKING!** Treatment includes: Bronchodilator drugs, antibiotics, lung transplantation, and alpha 1-proteinase inhibitors for some emphysema patients. However, those proteinase inhibitors are not recommended for those individuals who have developed emphysema as a result of cigarette smoking.

Recommendations & Suggestions: If you smoke cigarettes, or are in the process now of quitting, include these nutritives:

- Coenzyme Q-10 (Coenzyme Q-10) 100 Milligrams once daily
- EFA Essential Fatty Acids
- Vitamin E-800 IU's
- Beta Carotene-25,000 units (beta carotene is a precursor to vitamin A, as the body requires vitamin A, beta carotene will be transformed into Vitamin A).

- Vitamin C–1,000 milligrams, every four hours (not to exceed 3,000 milligrams daily)
- Deep breathing exercises and a brief walk in the fresh air.
- Avoid excessive amounts of red meat and mucous containing foods. I.e. milk, cheese, and other dairy products
- Add goat's milk, soy (rice and corn for protein)
- Meditation exercises

Eye Do's

by Eileen Renders N. D.   Copyright 1995

As we begin to mature, we become more subject to eye problems such as cataracts and/or decreased circulation to those arteries within the eye area, all of which can lead to surgery and/or loss of eyesight.

Taking a daily supplement of vitamin C can be helpful (preferably a natural form of vitamin C) and recent research at several universities now confirm that an enzyme (bilberry) extracted from the darkest of blue berries has been shown to be effective in enhancing the circulation to those tiny arteries that are responsible for providing nourishment and circulation to the eyes.

Once again, the essential fatty acids can also play a vital role, as they help to nourish and keep subtle all of the arteries which make up the Circulatory system.

Zinc also can be involved in helping to ward off eye problems, and it is therefore suggested that anyone suspecting that they may have a deficiency contemplate having a tissue hair analysis completed. Renders Wellness can provide such a service, and you will be given a color graph detailing normal ranges, your results and supplement recommendations with proper dosages. Corrections are also included for correcting any higher than normal ranges for such metals as lead, copper and aluminum.

Protect your eyes from the sun's rays with a good pair of protection sunglasses this year, and whenever operating garden machinery, wear appropriate safety glasses.

At the first sign of a sty, try some tea bags that have been brewed and cooled. They contain a fair source of tannic acid, which has been beneficial to many who have tried this remedy.

In order to keep the tear ducts functioning at high performance, use them! If you have nothing to cry about (and I do hope that is the case), try renting a sad video.

Eyes that are sporting many obvious broken blood vessels require immediate examination to determine the cause. High blood pressure, diabetes or conjunctivitis are a few of the possible culprits, though there are others.

Fatigue

by Eileen Renders N.D. Copyright 1997

Here is a subject which is often discussed, yet little understood. Probably this is because there are many underlying diseases and/or disorders associated with fatigue. This being true, we can then look at fatigue as more of a symptom than a disorder. And here is where it begins to become a little confusing, as there are simply so many problems associated with the fatigue symptom.

Proper diagnosis, therefore, will require the attention of a skilled and experienced practitioner, one who has available to him or her all of the up-to-the-minute tools of the diagnostic trade. At times, diagnosis may often require a process of elimination. To give you an idea as to the extent of the various common disorders linked with fatigue, consider the following; anemia, aortic stenosis, cirrhosis of the liver, colorectal cancer, depression, fibromyalgia, hepatitis, hyperthyroidism, menopause, mononucleosis and non-Hodgkin's disease to mention a few.

After ruling out many of the above disease, one might find that while they are relieved, they

69

are still in the dark as to why they are not feeling up to par, and that is the time to take a closer look at the stress level one is under and exactly how they are handling that stress. Poor nutrition, along with long standing deficiencies, could severely alter one's ability to carry out the process known as photosynthesis. That is when the body (through it's storage of proper nutrients and minerals) utilized the essential nutrients from the foods it is provided and converts them into energy. Some of the essential nutrients needed in order to accomplish this process are the essential fatty acids and chlorophyll. An improper diet full of refined white sugar, alcohol, etc. (Along with the effects of continued stress) can deplete our system of these essential nutrients, thus leading to fatigue and weakening of the immune system.

Hypotension (low blood pressure) and Epstein Barr virus have also been associated with Chronic Fatigue Syndrome. In the case of fibromyalgia and fatigue it should be known that there are presently no specific lab tests or X-Rays which can detect fibromyalgia. However, your doctor will base the diagnosis on your medical history, the identification of tender points, and the absence of other diseases. Describing the pain that you feel and where it is located, as clearly as you can, may help your doctor diagnose the problem.

Those suffering from diagnosed hypotension may consider including a bit of sodium chloride (table salt) into their diets. As most are aware, sodium chloride is the first substance individuals suffering form hypertension or high blood pressure are recommended to avoid.

For assistance in making your transition to a healthier lifestyle, contact your nearest Naturopath or Nutritionist.

Fats and Oils

by Eileen Renders N. D.   Copyright 1996

For the sake of those individuals who are interested in their health, but have not heard me speak about information revealed to us via Clinical Studies regarding the fats, may I repeat;

To begin with, there are three specific types of fats found in oils, *polyunsaturated, monounsaturated* and *saturated.* Of the three, polyunsaturated and the closely related monounsaturated are known as the *good fats.* It is, of course, the saturated fats which do us the most harm, or which are better known as the *bad fats.* Many oils contain toxic substances. Canola oil, for instance, contains Erucic acid. This is an acid which could ultimately effect many of the body's organs. One time containing as much as 40%Erucic acid (in the 1960's), new government standards allow canola oil to contain only 5% Erucic acid.

Caster oil contains 80 percent ricinoleic acid, and that is exactly whey the body attempts to eliminate this oil (along with everything else) in the intestines very quickly. Peanut oil may contain carcinogenic substances because they are grown in damp places, thus contaminated by fungus. These aflatoxin's found in peanuts are also found in corn. Aflatoxins may cause liver cancer. President Carter's brother Billy, who died of cancer, was thought by many to be cancer caused from high ingestion of peanuts. The Carter's lived and were raised in "Peanut country."

Cottonseed oil contains up to ½ percent of a cycloprene fatty acid that has a toxic effect on the liver and gallbladder. Heating of certain oils to high temperature produces free radicals, which at best age the body and at worst, damage the body. Vitamin E can protect the body's cell membranes from free-radical damage that takes place when oils are heated or become rancid.

Polyunsaturated fats are fats which are liquid and remain liquid. Sources are safflower oil, cottonseed oil, sunflower seeds, soy oil, primrose oil, corn oil, sesame oil, flax oil, and cod liver oil. Use only cold or expeller pressed oils, as when these oils are over-processed, they lose many of their benefits.

Monounsaturated oils (fats) include olive oil, avocado, canola, almonds, cashews, peanut and hazelnut. Because many of these fats (oils) may contain high portions of cholesterol, or in some way effect the blood cholesterol level, olive oil is the oil most preferred by the experts.

Fennel

by Eileen Renders N.D.

Copyright 1997

The Latin name for fennel is Foeniculum vulgare. Synonyms include fenkel, sweet fennel and wild fennel. Natural habitat is in most parts of Europe, but is indigenous to the shore of the Mediterranean, from whence it spreads eastward to India. It has followed civilization, especially where Italians have colonized. It is mainly comprised of a fixed oil, sugar mucilage and ash.

Pliny had much faith in its medicinal properties, claiming that it would cure 22 different diseases. Pliny also observed that serpents eat it when they cast off their old skins, and restore their sight by rubbing against it.

Fennel was used by Hippocrates and was also well-known to the ancient Egyptians. Down through the ages, this wonderful herb has been used in the treatment of many afflictions, such as failing sight, blindness, dropsy, adipose tissue, inflammations, fevers, nervous troubles and a score of many other conditions.

Fennel expels wind, provokes urine and is said to ease the pains of stones and help to break them. The FDA requires that all sausages manufactured within the United States must have fennel seed contained within, and that is because of fennel's known anti-viral, anti-bacterial properties. Hence, this makes fennel a good concoction for a winter tea or sore throat. Adding a wee bit of lemon only enhances its abilities. Due to its known abilities and value, it is said to contain sodium sulfate and probably some magnesium sulfate.

Leaves of Fennel have been used to garnish fish and sauces, soups and stews, while the root has been boiled as a vegetable. It has been used for young children for colic and is very soothing as a digestive aid. This herb has been used as an eyewash for sore or tired eyes.

FOLIC ACID   by Eileen Renders N. D.
Copyright Mar., 2001

Many of us may be aware that Folic acid is a water soluble vitamin, and an integral part of the B+complex vitamins. But, do most of us take in the recommended daily allotment? And do we understand the importance of this vital nutrient to our health?

#1- It is essential for the formation of healthy red blood cells and aids in the metabolism of protein.

#2 In conjunction with B-12 and vitamin-C, Folic Acid helps the body to produce *heme,* the Iron protein that is part of the hemoglobin, a requirement for the formation of red blood cells.

#3 - Folic acid is a carbon-carrier and recent studies show that *homocysteine* is a factor in the progression of both *atherosclerosis and osteoporosis, and has been shown to increase the risk of heart attack.* Clinical studies indicate that supplementation of folic acid actually lowers *homocysteine* levels in most individuals who fall within the high area of predetermined risk zone

Symptoms of Folic acid deficiency include; Shortness of breath, heart palpitations, nausea, weakness, irritability, headache and anemia.

Certain types of prescribed medications such as; Estrogens, alcohol, barbiturates, certain drugs used in chemotherapy (especially M*ethotrexate)* as well as the effects of excessive stress can interfere with the absorption of folic acid. There is no known toxicity associated with supplementation of folic acid; however, excessive intake can often disguise itself as a vitamin B-12 deficiency.

Folic acid as well as most vitamins should be taken in conjunction with other B vitamins.

The RDA (Recommended daily allotment   ) for adult females has been set at 180 micrograms, 200 micrograms for adult males, and slightly higher for pregnant and lactating females. The requirements for children vary and usually are set at 25 micrograms for babies 6 month and older, and 75 to 100 micrograms for children 6 to 10 years of age.

Note: This information and more can be found in FOOD ADDITIVES, NUTRIENTS AND SUPPLEMENTS A TO Z by Eileen Renders N. D..

Folic acid is found in the following types of foods;   Beans (1 cup)   160 to 350 Micrograms

Spinach, fresh, cooked (1 cup)   260 micrograms Oatmeal, fortified, instant (1-cup) 200 micrograms Asparagus, fresh cooked   Six spears 130 micrograms Peas, green (1 cup) 95 micrograms

Brussels sprouts (1 cup cooked)   95 micrograms Broccoli, chopped, cooked-1-cup 80 micrograms Corn, kernels (1 cup) 75 micrograms.

EXERCISE

For individuals who may want to exercise regularly, but are not sufficiently motivated, please consider the following Health benefits which are benefits of a regular Exercise routine:

~ Increases bone density, especially Walking, and "weight-bearing" exercises.

~ Stimulates the manufacture of hormones, which are required in order to optimally carry out normal internal processes.

~ It is a "Natural Stress Reliever", as it is known to release hormones (Endorphins, In particular) which reduce the Stress level.

~ It strengthens the Heart, which is a muscle (*"Use It, Or Lose It!"*), and helps to reduce the risk for Heart disease.

~ Lowers cholesterol (total blood lipid levels.)

~ Assists in helping to maintain proper weight, and management of the same.

~ Induces better sleep patterns.

~ Increases Metabolism.

~ Stimulates internal organs to perform better;

~ kidneys, bowels, heart, and etc. Thereby
reducing chances of constipation, water
retention, or heart disease!

~ Muscle weighs more than fat, and allows for a
higher caloric intake.

~ Enhances circulation, oxygen utilization,
thereby raising energy levels.

HEALTHIERFOOD CHOICES

By: Eileen Renders N. D. copyright 1999

More information on this subject can be found in "The Holistic Cookbook" by Eileen Renders 2001.

With the Holidays just around the corner we wanted share our Healthy Cheesecake recipe with you that you might savor the taste without sacrificing sound nutrition, or overloading with empty calories. .

Beverages; Mineral water, water, vegetable juices, or whole fruit juice made from pure concentrates. Caffeinated beverages rob the body of essential nutrients.

They also over-stimulate the Adrenal glands.

Breads; Whole grain, or multi grain breads. These breads usually are higher in nutritional value, and contain at least 2 grams of fiber per slice. And they do not contain saturated fats or dough conditioners.

Dairy Milk, yogurt, unprocessed cheeses;
Abundant in protein, Cottage cheese, goat cheese & etc. Calcium, and B-vitamins.

Fats;   Unsaturated varieties such as;   Sesame, Sunflower and Virgin Olive oil are ideal. It is recommended that hydrogenated oils are avoided, they include;   Palm kernel, and coconut oil, and cottonseed.

Fruits And Vegetables;   Fresh, or frozen (without heavy Creams) and are low in Sodium content hearty in Creams) with low sodium content will provide essential nutrients such as vitamins A, C, and the Bioflavonoids.

Vegetables;   Especially those dark green leafy varieties such as;   Broccoli, Spinach, Kale, Mustard greens or Turnips are an excellent source of vitamin K, and fat soluble chlorophyll. *Chlorophyll together with the EFA (Essential Fatty Acids) help to stimulate a process within the human body which is similar to the type of photosynthesis which occurs in nature.*

Flavonoids;   These are essential nutrients found in many species of fruits and vegetables and are necessary for the integrity of the arterial health, vision and other processes within the human body.

****

The Scoop On Garlic

By: Eileen Renders N. D.~ Copyright 1995

Garlic: medicinally speaking, Allium sativum. A member of the onion family, garlic has been cultivated in Egypt from earliest times, and was known in China more than two thousand years ago. Hippocrates used garlic to treat pneumonia and infected wounds. Garlic was used during the Great Plague in Europe, and during World War I in the treatment to Typhus and dysentery. Albert Schweitzer used garlic effectively against typhus, cholera and typhoid.

In 1992, at the American Chemical Society meeting in Washington, D.C., three Rutgers University researchers reported that chemicals in garlic may protect the liver from damage caused by large doses of the pain killer, acetaminophen, and may prevent the growth of lung tumors associated with tobacco smoke.

Garlic contains vitamins A, C and B1, as well as the minerals copper, iron, zinc, tin, calcium aluminum, sulphur, selenium and germanium.

It is absolutely known that garlic (organic sulfur) is a universal antiseptic. It's chemical constituents are: volatile oil (25%), mucilage (35%), albumin, sugar starch, fibrin and approximately 60% water. It has been used for everything from skin diseases to leprosy, and has been proven to be most beneficial (some experts say) in cases of small pox when applied to the soles of the feet in a linen cloth which was renewed daily. And even in such cases, it could soon be detected and strongly emitted from he breath.

ADVISABLE: *Renders Wellness* advises the use of garlic with the first signs of a cold or flu, along with about 1,000 mg. Of vitamin C.

CAUTION: Raw garlic when used in excess may cause anemia as well as various digestive problems, or could result in burns in the mouth, throat, esophagus and stomach.

RECOMMENDED: Dried, aged garlic...Kyolic. Garlic is best known for having effectively killed the germs that caused cholera and typhoid in the 1940's.

****

The Healing........Spirit

by Eileen Renders N.D. ~

How often have we heard it said; "He, or she gave up, and did not have the will to live any longer", and therefore, died? The spirit feeds the will, and in a sense might be connected with an energy force that lies deep within all of us. But, when that spirit is broken, the will to continue living on in this world is often shattered! And often following such a statement made regarding someone we have known, or may be related to, we often feel the need to clarify such a remark by explaining what it was (we believe) that cause that person to lose their will to live. Perhaps it was that this individual was ill for a very long period of time, and suffered much, yet found little encouragement. Maybe, that individual recently suffered the loss of a loved one which led to their loss of desire to live on without that person. Maybe, they were just lonely and weak, and stopped fighting, or exerting their will to live.

There are just as many reasons for such a lack of luster for live as there are individuals who succumb to the frailties of life as we have come to know it! But, the fact remains that the spirit is very connected to each individual's will. And without nurturing of that spirit, the will is weakened.

When there is no joy to life any longer, we are less likely to resist leaving this world behind! In fact, when negativities such as Anger, resentment, jealousy, hate, or even self-pity is able to consume one to the point that all sense of good is over-looked, our energies are virtually consumed by this negative energy of thought. Yet, life has also proven that those who have been given the sentence of death through diagnosis of a terminable disease have often beaten the odds. Common factors which surround this type of survivor often point to such strengths as;   Hope, faith, love of life, and a quiet determination to continue on his/her journey living each day as it is dealt to them, and without dwelling upon death. Negative energies such as resentment, anger, or any of the others often consume one to the point that it can rob vital nutrients from the body, helping to squeeze the life out of a body that could be ill, or deprived.

Therefore, regardless of one's physical or emotional problems, it is a positive decision to spend one's energy and time here on Earth wisely by concentrating on positive thoughts which lead to positive feelings (emotions), and/or actions!

Spend this Holiday season in gratefulness for your good health by helping those who are elderly, ill, or handicapped. Invite them to dinner, or stop by and bring them something made with love.

****

Have A Heart

by Eileen Renders N. D.   Copyright 1995

It's the time of the year when our heart's and our thoughts are turned toward our loved ones. Have you ever wondered why we express love as coming from the heart? We accept this to be true by confirming the fact that we have often been known to say; "If you don't return by love, my heart will simply break!"

Perhaps we can now all agree on at least one level; our feelings and emotions definitely can either have a positive or a negative effect upon our health. Regardless of whether you are now in love or in search of a new love, it will pay off if you take care of your heart!

In keeping with this month's "Sweetheart" theme, we offer the following information for those who are interested in securing your heart's health.

1. For adequate oxygen and circulation benefits, exercise (with your doctor's approval) and take daily supplements of cayenne capsules to help the body "Break up" any excess accumulation of fibrin, the clotting factor, which

keeps us from bleeding extensively when cut, but which can also accumulate to excess in some individuals who are sedentary or nutritionally deficient. Excess fibrin is what is often responsible for clot formation and is involved in strokes.

2. Refrain from cigarettes, excess alcohol and coffee.

3. Remember to get adequate amounts of the essential fatty acids, linolenic and the linoleic acids. While their benefits are too numerous to mention here, they can be of aid in helping reduce the risk of arteriosclerosis or hardening of the arteries.

4. Limit the amount of saturated fats in the diet to no more than 20% Fifteen percent is the ideal number according to many nutritional experts, and a figure to which I am inclined to agree.

5. Avoid toxic chemicals, many of which are known to be carcinogens such as those found in foods (and I use the word loosely here) containing food preservatives, food additives and food dyes. They are most often found in boxes, bags and cans

6.   Refrain from excess consumption of red meats, which contain saturated fats and often synthetic hormones, all of which can add to unwanted pounds and over stimulation with these hormones which may be linked to certain types of heart disease.

7.   Take a daily supplement of Co-Enzyme Q-10 (a 30 milligram strength) with lots of fresh fruits and vegetables.

8.   If you cannot exercise, consider Guided Imagery or Visualization as a way in which to reduce stress and for boosting one's immune system.

For your consideration: A tissue hair analysis, which will test your body for 36 minerals and six toxins to assure that you have adequate amounts of Calcium, Magnesium, Copper, etc. and that you do not show an overload of certain other minerals which, in high percentages, may cause serious health problems. For instance: too little copper is often associated with a high risk of heart attack, too little selenium, on the other hand might be an indication that there is insufficient antioxidant protection against free radicals.

Diabetes/Beneficial Herbs and Nutrients

by Eileen Renders N.D.   Copyright 1999

Sugar cravings have been linked, according to many nutritional experts, to the body's attempt to restore and/or maintain adequate serotonin levels. The unsaturated fats (essential fatty acids ~ linoleic and linolenic acids) assist the body to stimulate the production and uptake of serotonin, thus leading to a clear mind, and sense of well being. **Vitamin-B6** (part of the B complex vitamin) can also assist in alleviating sugar cravings. Rather than supplementing this vitamin alone, it should be taken in combination with a B+complex vitamin in order to eliminate other B vitamin imbalances. 100 Milligrams is a suggested dose.

Chromium picolinate~ Employed by insulin, chromium assists cells to better utilize glucose, and a deficiency in this element raises the body's requirement for insulin. And since insulin contributes to the body's excretion of chromium, diabetics dependent on insulin injections often have a pronounced Chromium deficiency.

Fenugreek~ *Trigonella foenum-graceum* This herb dates back as far as Hippocrates. Egyptian women regarded it as an aid in easing the pain associated with childbirth, and it was often recommended to nursing mothers to insure a healthy supply of milk. Containing mucilage, saponins, alkaloids, protein, vitamins and minerals, Western researchers have found this herb to have a "hypoglycemic" effect. In some studies using urine samples, it was shown to cut in half existing sugar levels.

Ginseng~ Chinese pharmacology indicates that this herb has been shown in Laboratory studies (with animals) to stimulate the release of insulin from the pancreas, and can also support adrenal gland function.

Vitamin E~ This potent antioxidant assists the body in better insulin reaction, and is therefore beneficial to diabetics. Vitamin E may help in preventing cardiovascular disease, secondary to diabetes.

Zinc~ A mineral which assists in regulation of the body's energy supply, it is one of the substances which comprise what constitutes the hormone insulin.

Sugar substitute~ An herb known as Stevia for your daily cup (one) of coffee. Remember that Aspartame, and various other sugar substitutes are on the "Suspect" list of carcinogens, as is caffeine.

****

HIV/AIDS

by Eileen Renders N.D.   Copyright 1999

As a practicing Herbalist since 1995, I was fortunate to become involved in a program funded by the N.I.H. (National Institutes of Health) which was the result of a five year Study by the National Institutes of Health, Bethesda, MD. Into the possible benefit to be derived by the HIV/AIDS populations through Consultations with an Herbalist with a degree. That Contract ran three years, until RENDERS WELLNESS declined an extended Contract due to a cut in the Services "Allowed." Still involved with the HIV/AIDS diagnosed individuals, we provide Nutritional education, including a reference resource for those foods which are considered "Antagonistic" to optimum wellness. . Detoxification (for protection of the Liver, especially when potent prescribed medications are selected course), and proven herbal recommendations for Immune enhancement.

Following are several suggestions which have proven beneficial to those HIV/AIDS diagnosed individuals who have participated in the Renders Wellness Program;

Ascorbic Acid (natural form of Vitamin-C) 1/4 tsp. Four times a day= 2,000 Milligrams, St. John's wort Extract, CO-Enzyme-Q-10 (60 milligrams - once daily), Grapeseed Extract (also helps to maintain proper ph, and thus prevent Thrush), Tumeric, B+ Complex vitamin (100 Milligrams ~ in addition to Multi vitamin), The Chinese herb Astragalus Root Extract ~ 15 drops per day, Selenium (100 micrograms), Soy, Pectin, and avoidance of the following;

Alcohol, refined white sugar (an acid which causes an acidic internal environment which opens the door to Candida), refined white flour, caffeine, hydrogenated oils, fried foods, excess amounts of red meat, high fat foods, nitrates and nitrates which transform into "nitrosamines" in the stomach and are known carcinogens.

Note: While Renders Wellness believed in natural therapies, and in fact, assisted individuals diagnosed HIV/AIDS AS A nutritional and Herbal Consultant subcontracted through THE ATLANTIC CITY MEDICAL CENTER in Atlantic

City, it has always been considered "Complimentary" or "Adjuvant" Services. Yet, Renders Wellness found that in conclusion of this Program, we had been providing more than services. This discovery was made in part, when several HIV individuals participating in the Program (Funded by the N.I.H.) found that their body could not withstand the potent side effects of such drugs as AZT, and removed themselves voluntarily from the ingesting of these drugs.

It was only then, that Renders Wellness was able to witness firsthand, the astonishing benefits associated with simply the nutritional support of Consultations with only herbal recommendations which were enhancing the Immune system, without the antagonistic effects of potent toxic drugs.

Ironically, in February of 2001, The Herald Tribune Newspaper reported that the AIDS panel had reviewed their long held policy and guidelines for treating HIV/AIDS by "Hitting hard and Fast" as a recommendation which brought with it, increased concerns over the toxic effects of such therapies. In fact, they revised their approach of "Hit early, hit hard", and recommended that treatment should be delayed in individuals without symptoms!

HEALTH NOTES

by; Eileen Renders N. D.

Copyright 4-2000

Fact: *Recent studies have released results which indicate that individuals who are taking ACE Inhibitors to treat CAD Cardiovascular disease may be at an estimated 28% higher risk for developing adult diabetes.*

Fact: *Due to serious side effects, at least five (5) drugs previously used for treating Asthma have been recalled. Check with your pharmacist to find out which ones are included, and check the names on your own drug for treating Asthma.*

Note: *Some prescriptions prescribed for treating high blood lipid levels can cause; Muscle weakness (report this sign to your Dr. immediately), and Liver disorders.*

Fact; *One of the leading causes of heart disease (including heart-attack and/or Stroke) are vascular disorders. In fact, hardening of the arteries (Arteriosclerosis) has little to do with high cholesterol levels, and Atherosclerosis (cholesterol, or plaque build up) are disorders* *which can be addressed nutritionally, lessening*

the risk of a Cardiovascular event.

Postscript;   *See your personal*

Nutritionist/Herbalist soon!

HYPERALDOSTERONISM

by Eileen Renders N. D.

Copyright Mar 2000

Primary (Conn's syndrome) is uncommon in 70% of patients, and usually is the result of a benign aldosterone-producing adrenal adenoma. A disorder more often associated with women (at least 3 times more prevalent in women than in men) and often strikes an individual between the ages of 30 to 50. In 15% to 30% of patients with primary aldosteronism, the cause is unknown, however while it is rare, the cause can be pinpointed as "adrenalcortical *hyperplasia* (in children), or carcinoma.

In primary hyperaldosteronism, chronic aldosterone (often better known as the Oight or flight" hormone) excess is completely independent of the renin-angiotensin system and, as a matter of fact, it suppresses plasma renin activity. This aldosterone (hormone released from the Adrenal glands) excess heightens sodium reabsorption by the kidneys which leads to hypernatremia (a presence in the blood of an abnormally high content of sodium) and simultaneously, hypokalemia (the presence of abnormally low serum potassium in the blood) with an increased extra cellular fluid volume.

Expansion of intravascular fluid volume also occurs and results in what is known as "Volume dependent hypertension" a condition which causes an increased cardiac output, or heart strain.

Secondary hyperaldosteronism ~ A similar condition as primary hyperaldosteronism with much of the same symptoms, secondary hyperaldosteronism however, refers to a type of condition whereas a"Cause" (and quite possibly, therefore a "Cure" can be effected) has been detected. There are several, including a combination of a couple of causes which are most common to secondary hyperaldosteronism, and they are as follows; A. Renal artery stenosis (extra-adrenal pathology) B. Wilm's tumor C. Oral contraceptives D. Various disorders unrelated to hypertension.

Signs and symptoms ~ These symptoms may be experienced alone, or in combination with others, and they are as follows; (A.) Hypokalemia (Diabetes due to hypokalemia) (B). Muscle

weakness (C). Fatigue (D). Headaches (E).
Paresthesia (a tingling sensation often described as
pins and needles (F.) Hypertension (G.) Edema.
Diagnosis ~ The following signs help your
physician to make a diagnosis, along with one=s
medical history;

1. Low serum potassium levels in an individual
    who is NOT taking diuretics, or who shows
    no signs of edema.
2. Higher than "normal" serum bicarbonate
3. High urinary aldosterone levels.
4. Increased (as much as 30 to 50%) in plasma
    volume.

Note: Often misdiagnosed as hypertension, or
Being treated as hypertension, without finding the
Underlying cause!

5.   Renal angiography

Treatment ~ If a tumor is found, an
Adrenalectomy will be recommended. The
Associative condition of hypertension must also be
addressed with a "Potassium sparing" diuretic.
Sodium restriction is strongly advised. And be

advised that there is a Laboratory test known as a "Suppression Test" which can be carried out which can make for a clearer determination by your physician as to whether or not, your hyperaldosteronism is primary, or secondary, and therefore be better able to move forward with proper treatment.

Foods high in potassium include; Sunflower seeds, potatoes, bananas, dairy products (cheese), artichokes, meats, poultry, fish, garlic, Brewer's yeast, oranges, and most vegetables.

RENDERS WELLNESS or any Nutritional Therapist will help to provide support, along with natural diuretics in order to maintain normal blood volume which alleviates secondary hypertension.

Other Foods high in potassium include; Bananas oranges, whole grains, Sunflower seeds Mint Leaves, potatoes, meats, poultry, fish, legumes, nuts, Garlic, Brewer's yeast, avocados, raisins, dairy products, including cheese and yogurt! Kiwi, parsley, beets, watercress, artichokes, celery root, plantains, kelp, and wheatgrass.

Natural "Potassium sparing" diuretics

Cornsilk (the herb)

parsley

kelp

yogurt

pumpkin and/or squash seeds

kiwis (both a good source for potassium (over 250 milligrams each) and other beneficial Natural diuretic!

Hyperactivity *and Ritalin*

By; Eileen Renders N. D.

Attention deficit hyperactive disorder is the medical term given to children who are considered hyperactive. While it is a disorder more prevalent in children, it has been diagnosed in older children, and some adults. Symptoms range from mild to severe, and include: Motor skills, memory problems, and/or language difficulties. The demonstrated "Problems" often associated with these children, should in no way be considered indicative of a child's intelligence, for many are found to be above average in intelligence upon proper Testing.

The possible causes for this disorder are many; some of these causes may include: Emotional stress, an inability to interpret incoming information adequately, sleep disorders, hearing loss, prenatal drug abuse, food additives, lead poisoning, certain medicines and perhaps many other undiscovered possibilities.

A disorder which affects teachers, and the classroom, the hyperactive child often will display behavioral problems such as: impulsiveness, mood swings, or unmanageableness, including and inability to adhere to rules.

Although these children basically want to confirm, or "fit-in", much like the rest of his or her peers, and ability to exert control over his or her irrational spurts of energy, often appear to the child, to be impossible. This feeling of failure to the child, often carries a heavy burden of guilt and sorrow, and can leave the child feeling isolated, strange, or different from his or her classmates.

Treatment for this disorder should first include medical testing which would rule out causes such as visual or hearing problems, or neurological disabilities.

Drugs used to treat hyperactivity include: Premoline, Dextroamphetamine (Dexedrine), Thiordazine, Tricyclic antidepressant medications and Methylphenidate (Ritalin). The drug of choice for this disorder is often Ritalin. Ritalin is a stimulant which has proven to be effective as a stimulant, but is somewhat calming to the central nervous system.

Potential side effects of this drug include the following: decreased appetite, weight loss, retarded growth, irritability, increased heart rate, and or blood pressure.

From a nutritional viewpoint: Some studies have shown that these children may be reacting to an excess of iodine, which could be the result of high intake of salty foods. Many junk, or snack foods that contain high sodium chloride (including iodine) are the favorite snack foods of many children: potato chips, pretzels, French fries, peanuts, canned soups, and many other types of snack foods.

Another factor involved with most hyperactive children is the possibility of a nutritional deficiency, and/or other imbalances due to inadequate nutrition, or an impaired digestive system. Many children diagnosed ADHD are also hyper-sensitive to such Food Additives, or Food Preservatives as;   Food Colorings, MSG (a preservatives once often found in Chinese Take-Out foods, and others), hydrogenated oils, and other chemicals, including sugar substitutes such as those often found in diet sodas, and other foods and/or beverages.

Refined white sugar can be considered an antagonist, especially when it is consumed in excess, as it interferes with the body's ability to make available the essential B+ Complex vitamins. Refined white sugar (in excess) can cause an immediate burst of energy due to the secretion of insulin into the blood stream, but will be followed by a quick fall. Over production of insulin can lead to obesity because when we put out more insulin that the body can immediately utilize as energy, the balance is stored in the body as fat.

These suggestions are "Natural Therapeutics", and include;

1.   Placing the child on a fresh "whole food" diet of fresh fruits and vegetables (with adequate amounts of protein and whole grains, of course.) Elimination of Soda, Aspartame (or any sugar substitute), high Sodium Chloride snack foods, junk foods in general, hydrogenated oils (such as Palm kernel, Coconut & etc., red dyes and yellow dyes, and blue dyes often an ingredient found in candy bars.

2.   Replacing junk foods with more nutritional choices, including;   Home-made muffins, low Sodium pretzels, yogurt, applesauce, and fresh fruits. ~ Provide encouragement, emotional support, understanding, and lots of LOVE!

3.   The herb Kava together with the herb Lemon balm is a mild brain stimulant, but also works to calm the body. Doses should be minimal, and a visit to your local Nutritionist/Herbalist will provide proper dose recommendations according to your child's age, weight and etc

4.   A multiple vitamin is recommended, and should be given according to age.

5.   Teaching your child the benefits of self-control is essential, and setting priorities will help him/her to maintain proper balance between Schoolwork, Nutrition, Play and Rest.

6.   It is strongly recommended that you have a Mineral   Hair Analysis (usually taken at your N.D.'S Office) done to determine whether or not, your child has high tissue levels of one, or more of the toxic metals;   Lead, Arsenic, Mercury, Lead and etc. NOTE: A Tissue Mineral Hair Analysis is a Laboratory Test that is completed in a Laboratory Licensed to perform same, and is registered within the State it operates, and has become a mainstay test being utilized by none other than The New York City's finest men in blue, their Policemen.

Note: Uncovering any high concentrations of toxic minerals such as: Lead, Aluminum, Mercury and etc. calls for immediate attention (Oral chelation) as these toxic levels not only interfere with neurotransmitter performance, but could eventually lead to other neurological problems!

****

Iron Deficiency & (Restless Legs Syndrome)

by Eileen Renders N.D. ~
Copyright Nov., 1999

While RLS (Restless Legs Syndrome) seems to be becoming more common than once was, there is still little research being done to pinpoint a cause. Restless legs syndrome, or periodic limb movements PLM is more common in people over the age of 65. In fact, it is said that as much as 50% of the elderly experience this symptom to some degree. A disorder which usually happens during the night, it can be a mild disorder which occurs infrequently, or can occur as much as a couple of times per minute, contributing to a sleep disorder. Of those effected, only about 40% or so will experience it as having a detrimental effect upon their everyday lives. Severe cases of course, are often plagued with insomnia, and sleep deprivation may negatively impact one's daily life.

Some findings indicate that Selenium is often associated with some types of muscular complaints, and magnesium often is all that is required for alleviating muscle cramps often referred to as a "Charlie horse." When a magnesium deficiency exists for a continued period of time, calcium deposits can accumulate in the joints of the bones, resulting in Osteoporosis. And when excessive amounts of calcium is present in large amounts, it not only builds up in the tissues of the ligaments and tendons. The first studies ever done regarding RLS date as far back as thirty years ago. The reason for that study was the fact that a definite correlation between Restless Legs Syndrome and a low Iron levels had been noted. Ironically, although this clinical finding has been documented more than thirty years ago, ongoing studies were halted. More recently however, researchers at the Dept. of Geriatric Medicine of the Royal Liverpool University in Liverpool, U.K. did initiate just such a study using approximately 18 to 20 subjects in both patients and controls, all were over sixty years of age.

Reported findings showed serum ferritin levels were lower in patients with RLS in comparison to control subjects. At the same time, it was noted that the following nutritional levels did not differ between both groups studied; B-12, Folic acid, hemoglobin, and serum iron. In order to draw a significant conclusion, the researchers used a scale of 1 to 10 in order to rate the intensity of symptoms described by those patients diagnosed with Restless Legs Syndrome. In the final analysis, researchers found that the severity of each patient's symptoms directly corresponded to the lower levels of serum ferritin found in each patient.

Conclusion: Fifteen patients with RLS were given 200 milligrams of ferrous sulfate three times a day for eight weeks. Each patient's ferritin level was improved from 1 point to 4 points, which directly corresponded to how low their initial ferritin levels were. All patient's symptoms improved markedly regardless of whether or not, the Iron deficiency was accompanied by anemia.

Note: It is important to remember that high intake of the minerals Calcium, Magnesium and Zinc can have a negative effect upon the body's ability to properly absorb Iron. Anti-inflammatory drugs such as aspirin and ibuprofen may also lead to iron loss through gastrointestinal bleeding.　Vitamin C on the other hand, contributes to the absorption of Iron.　After having said all of the above, this article would provide little help were it not to include the following remark;

Balance is the goal in order to promote internal harmony, and "More is never better!"　High levels of iron could increase one's risk of a heart disease by promoting entry of free radicals into the blood stream which can damage the walls of the arteries.

Vitamins C, and E are strong antioxidants, and help prevent oxidative damage triggered by high levels of iron.

LECITHIN AND ATHEROSCLEROSIS

by: *Eileen Renders N. D.*

Copyright Aug., 2000

A disease marked by fatty deposits within the artery walls, these fatty deposits eventually develop into plaque which causes obstruction of blood flow.

As far back as the middle fifties, renown Nutritionist Adele Davis provided insight into this disease (backed up by Scientific research) which explains how Lecithin, a nutrient made by the body, but only when sufficient amounts of specific B-vitamins are available in the body (such as B-6, Choline, and Inositol) helps to break down cholesterol into tiny particles which are able then to pass through the bodys tissues.   Only when we are deficient in Lecithin does cholesterol become large, thus getting trapped in the blood and arterial walls.

Cholesterol deposits interfere with how oxygen is supplied to the brain.   Lowering blood cholesterol increases the oxygen supply and speeds recovery!   Lecithin contains;   Fat, Choline, Inositol and unsaturated fats.   Vitamin

B-6 along with Magnesium assist the body in making lecithin. To insure sufficient amounts of Inositol, Choline and Linoleic acid (those essential nutrients which help to maintain optimum transport and functioning of human cells, (especially when high blood cholesterol levels and/or Atherosclerosis has been diagnosed) is to supplement daily with Lecithin made only from pure Soy granules. Lecithin made from pure Soy granules is an excellent source for Inositol, Choline and Linoleic acid.

Foods to limit or avoid include; Hydrogenated oils such as; Palm kernel oil, Coconut, Peanut & etc. Hydrogenated oils deplete the body's supply of the good fatty acids such as Linoleic acid. Nitrites and nitrates such as those found in Hot dogs, luncheon meats, bacon and other smoked meats. Nitrites and nitrates are known to form a dangerous cancer-causing compound known as nitrosamines when they are combined with digestive juices. Also, while protein is an important part of nutrition, the amount of saturated fat intake should be limited.

Legionnaires Disease

by; Eileen Renders N. D.   Copyright 1998

Legionnaires's disease has been described as an acute bronchopneumonia produced by a discriminating gram-negative bacillus. This disease first became known in 1976 when 182 people became severely ill at an American Legion convention in Philadelphia. Twenty nine of those individuals later died. A disease that may occur epidemically, or individually, it can be accompanied by pneumonitis, and carries a mortality rate of 15%.

From that fateful episode, we have found what caused that epidemic and we now know who is most susceptible and how we can best avoid such an episode.

Signs and symptoms include fatigue, diarrhea, anorexia, headache, chills, and a fever which develops within 12-48 hours. Some patients have demonstrated other symptoms such as nausea, vomiting, disorientation, chest pain, mental confusion, and 50% of patients develop bradycardia (a slowing of the heart beat to less than 50 beats per minute)

Treatment usually includes an antibiotic treatment as soon as diagnosis has been made and the patient is encouraged to practice deep breathing techniques in order to excrete toxins. Close monitoring of vital signs is recommended, and the patient is usually made comfortable climatically, with good ventilation.

If you live in a large house which has been made airtight to conserve energy in the winter, and you have an air-conditioning vent system which has never been professionally cleaned by a company that specializes in this type of cleaning, you could be a risk for breeding gram-negative bacillus. And when the cooling system goes on one year - bingo! This bacteria could be forced into your home's breathing air. This bacteria is uncommon in a system which is new, or could be rare in a home which is not so air tight that ventilation is prohibited. Still, it might be a good idea to consider the costs of such a service, verses the risk potentially possible with NOT taking such precautions. Remember this was *not a disease of such epidemic form, prior to the invention of central air-conditioning being installed into*

commercial, industrial, and residential buildings.
While many residences and/or commercial sites may require this type of service on a regular basis (such as Restaurants in High rise buildings), perhaps that is not the case with your home. Determining factors include;   Ventilation (or air circulation quality), number of floors, and heat and cooking exhaust systems.   To remain on the side of Safety, a professional evaluation by a reputable Company specializing in the cleaning of Exhaust systems

---

Lemon Verbena *Aloysia triphylla* ~

by Eileen Renders N.D.   Copyright 1999

The flowering tops and the leaf itself are the parts used, and contain mainly *Flavonoids and Volatile oils.* In foods, Lemon Verbena has traditionally been used in alcoholic beverages and in herbal teas.

Pharmaceutical comment confirms that uses for this herb are attributable to its volatile oil content, and more specifically; its flavone constituents. That is the opinion at least, of the contributors of a specific publication offered by The Pharmaceutical Press.

Lemon Verbena has been given the GRAS stamp which translates to mean; *Generally Regarded As Safe* by the FDA, Food And Drug Association.

Herbal use for Lemon verbena has been recommended by Herbalists for years for relief of such ailments as;   Antispasmodic, colds, as a sedative, and most beneficially for Asthmatics.

Side effects   There have been no recorded side effects documented for Lemon verbena, however due to its Terpene content as a volatile oil, it could be regarded as an irritant capable of being strong enough to cause kidney irritation if improperly used; ***Including improper dose, or in instances of prolonged use.***

Contraindications: Individuals who are pregnant, nursing, or with diagnosed kidney problems would be advised to avoid Lemon verbena.

Recommendations: For maximum benefit, without risk for potential harm, Herbal teas containing Lemon verbena is recommended. The diluted tea is safe, and can therefore, be taken several times a day.

****

More Natural Cholesterol-Lowering Remedies (Lipids)

by Eileen Renders N.D. ~ Copyright 1999

Before considering resorting to prescribed drugs for the purpose of lowering one's blood lipid levels, it would be wise to be aware that these drugs can often lead to a Liver toxicity, especially for those individuals who may already be suffering from a diagnosed Liver problem, women who may be pregnant, or nursing, and possibly those with various other medically diagnosed disorders.   Others who appear to have healthy Livers must still have regular Liver function tests done under the supervision of their physician. *Yet how many patients (especially the middle-aged, or elderly)* are aware that by the time we reach middle age, the Liver is only capable of operating at approximately 45 to 55% capacity as it once did when we were twenty

years of age?   Ironically, it is at just that age (middle age) when many patients are prescribed not one, not two, but three, four, or five prescribed drugs!   Then, we cannot lose sight of the cost of these drugs, many of which cost as much as three dollars each, making a 30 day supply $90.00 or more. Others considerations are; Risk factors, i.e.; Diabetes, obesity, stress, cigarette smoking, sedentary lifestyles, Inherited tendencies, and poor nutrition. Elevated cholesterol readings alone, cannot be totally relied upon as accessing one's risk for Heart disease, or Stroke. And that is exactly why The American Heart Association as provided a Ratio for increased risk for heart disease based upon the number arrived at, after dividing the LDL (bad cholesterol) number by the HDL (good cholesterol) number. **Before you resort, or submit to prescribed drugs, try these natural, and effective remedies;**

A Carrot a day.

More fiber.

Decreased consumption of fats and sugars.

More fruit

If you have not been successful after 60 days, include one of the following Supplements;

Pectin ~ A concentrated substance extracted from fruits, but be careful, it can cause Constipation.

Psyllium husk ~ Fiber

*Vanadyl sulfate ~ **Caution:** Use only as recommended on bottle, and limit dose to once a day!*

Manganese~ 5 to 10 Milligrams daily

Vitamin C ~ 1,000 Milligrams a day

Garlic oil capsules ~ 1,000 Milligrams a day

Tumeric ~ 1,000 Milligrams a day (also a very beneficial Antioxidant) This Indian spice travels through the bloodstream, and like a magnet, picks up the fat in the blood, and escorts it out!

Red Yeast Rice ~ 600 Milligrams taken once a day, preferably at bedtime for maximum effectiveness.

****

LYMPHATIC SYSTEM

by Eileen Renders N.D. Copyright 1998

Understanding exactly what the "Lymph System" is, and how it functions can better enable us on how to better protect the health of this valuable internal system. That is, to the best of each individual's ability. The Lymphatic system involves *lymph nodes, lymphatic vessels,* and lymphatic organs which include the *tonsils, thymus,* and the *spleen.* The thymus is a gland with a double-duty function and responsibility. It works in conjunction with various other aspects of the **endocrine system**, and of course, as a vital part of the **lymphatic system.**

However, rather than carrying blood, the lymphatic vessels contain a watery fluid which is whitish in color, along with lymphocytes (white blood cells involved in the body"s Immune system), proteins and a portion of fatty molecules (a molecule is described as the smallest particle of an element, or compound that can exist in the free state and yet still retain the characteristics of the element or compound it represents.) The lymph fluid differs greatly from the circulatory system in

126

that it does not circulate continuously through a selected group of vessels, and it does not have a pump. The lymph fluid is circulated through the lymphatic vessels with a destination which eventually enters back into the circulatory system, and does so by passing through the large ducts, such as the **thoracic duct.** Groupings of lymph nodes can be noticed in the axillary (armpit) and in the inguinal (groin) areas of the body. The lymph system has several functions, one of which is to move the fluids, and other large molecules from the tissue cavities which accumulate around cell sites. Moving them, and other fat-related nutrients from the digestive tract back into the blood stream. And the lymphatic system is also responsible for maintaining healthy functioning of the *Immune System,* a critical part of our defense mechanism of the body as we fight off invaders or disease.

What can go wrong with the lymph system? As children, we are constantly cleansing the lymph system through child-like activities such as jumping rope, a game of catch-tag, or skating, or whatever. It is the constant, or consistent up and down movements which push the lymph fluid through the vessels, easily and thoroughly accomplishing the task it was meant to do. Playing real hard, and then drinking as much water as an empty gas tank is another way we keep things **moving along efficiently.** But as we begin to age, or are more apt to become sedentary, our lymph system may not perform for us as it was once capable of performing. And when that occurs, the fluid and molecules can begin to build up, and sort of stagnate, clogging up the lymph system, and leaving us much more vulnerable to free radicals. So, if you are over 40, and not up to jumping rope this Saturday morning, perhaps just a brisk walk for twenty minutes will be enough to do the trick!

Marika Von Viczay, a Naturopathic physician and director of the ISIS Health and Rejuvenation Center in Asheville, North Carolina states that when lymphatic circulation slows down, or becomes impaired, the system becomes toxic. And for those who cannot tolerate physical exercise because of health conditions, or are bed ridden, she emphasizes the benefit of a **light**

massage on the exit points of the subclavian vein where the lymph enters and this breaks up stagnation.

Caution: It must be emphasized however, and according to Viczay, "To over stimulate, or to deeply massage this area of the subclavian vein would be counter productive, as it could do more harm than good!" **Note:** *It is also important to make certain that one is consuming adequate amounts of antioxidants, such as beta-carotene, selenium, zinc, and vitamin C. Insure also, that the diet includes Carrots, whole grains, seeds, and adequate amounts of water.*

Macular degeneration

by Eileen Renders   Copyright 1999

While there are a couple of types of Macular degeneration, one type is slow progressing, and can cause up to 20% of central vision loss in about five years. The more serious of the two types can progress rapidly, and is said to be responsible for nearly 12% of blindness in the United States, and almost 17% of newly diagnosed cases of blindness each year. Both types are considered to be age related, and without any predisposing conditions. It is however, the result of hardening and obstruction of the retinal arteries, and are common to degenerative changes which occur in the elderly. **Diagnosis** is generally made through what is known as *Indirect ophthalmoscopy, or fundus examination through a dilated pupil.* Another comparative test is the *I.V. fluorescein angiography which is a sequence of photographs which can pinpoint leaking vessels. Fluorescein dye runs into the tissues beginning at the subretinal neovascular net.* Another test known as *Amsler's grid will show the total visual field loss.*

Bilberry~ 50 milligram Extract/25% Anthocyanosides

Recommendation: Three capsules once daily. Should constipation occur, eliminate one capsule a day.

Lutein~ Spinach, or lutein based antioxidants may not only slow progression of certain types of Macular degeneration, but may gradually reverse failing vision. According to Stuart Richer, O.D., Ph.D., at the North Chicago VA Medical Center, and who is chief of the optometry department, "Lutein may be the key." It seems, as Richer explains; "This carotenoid accumulates in the retina and prevents cells from dying off in the center. Lutein is converted to zeaxanthin, an isomer that blocks blue and ultraviolet radiation. Zeaxanthin also functions as a single oxygen quencher, much like beta-carotene. In the macula, these carotenoids are referred to as macular pigment." Dr. Richer advises pharmacists to recommend a lutein based antioxidant complex, and that people with ARMD (Age Related Macular Degeneration) eat spinach, and take a vitamin E supplement.

Vitamin C~ 500 milligrams ~ taken three times a day. Vitamin C is a water soluble vitamin, and the body will release that which it cannot immediately utilize. Breaking up dose will help the body to optimally benefit from a 1500 milligram intake.

Vitamin E~ 400 I.U.'s daily. This is usually one capsule.

Note: Individuals who are prone to high blood pressure, or who may hyper-sensitive to vitamin-E could experience elevated blood pressure when more than 400 I.U.'s a day are ingested.

Zinc~ An antioxidant mineral, 30 milligrams a day will help to combat free radicals, which are in part, responsible for many eye disorders.

****

Magnesium

by Eileen Renders N.D.

Copyright 1996

Magnesium is an "Essential" mineral. Approximately 25 grams are present in an adult. Half of that amount is contained in the bones with the remainder found in the various soft tissues throughout the body. Some of the locations where the highest concentrations are found are in the muscles (including the heart), the skeletal muscles, the liver and the pancreas. It is a key element for cellular metabolism. It assists the body in stimulating the many enzyme reactions which must occur.

Yet, emotional stress and alcohol consumption are just two of the many ways in which we can lose this mineral. Physical exercise such as skiing, bicycling and running are other ways in which a loss can occur. Pregnant women or breast feeding mothers, infants and individuals on certain medications are often vulnerable to a shortage of this critical mineral.

Some of the body's symptoms which might be indicative of a shortage could be associated with some of the following: anxiousness, irritability (magnesium is one of the body's natural sedatives), excessive perspiration, muscle cramps, certain types of hypertension, constipation, arthritis and more.

Magnesium needs to be in a relative balanced proportion with calcium, or it could trigger other symptoms and problems (that's another column).

The adrenal gland secretes a hormone called aldosterone, and this hormone adjusts the rate at which magnesium is excreted through the kidneys. Losses tend to increase with the use of diuretics and with the consumption of alcohol, as stated earlier.

Magnesium can be found in milk, figs, fresh greens, fish and sea foods, tofu, black strap molasses, apples, kelp, soybeans, wheat germ, oatmeal, apricots and brewer's yeast.

Menopause

By: Eileen Renders N. D. Copyright 1998

In recent years there has been an overwhelming response from women who are approaching mid-life for Alternative remedies that will address the annoying symptoms associated with menopause. It has been suggested that women who belong to a family where Cancer is prevalent, could place themselves at an increased risk for Cancer themselves by taking any form of Estrogen replacement drugs. Estrogen has been linked to Cancer because it has been shown to not only contribute to the disease, but to "Feed it once it has shown its presence.

Symptoms often associated with menopause include insomnia, nightly sweats, and spontaneous flushing of the skin. After menopause, women are shown to be more susceptible to more serious disorders such as; *Heart disease, osteoporosis, and high blood lipid levels.*

Phytochemicals, and **Phytohormones** are chemicals and hormones derived from Plants. They are organic (as are our bodies), therefore often more compatible with the human body, in that they are more readily metabolized, and utilized. "Phyto" means plant. While these phytohormones are plant foods, roots, or the like, and really do not contain hormones, they do provide a unique ability for *"balancing, and/or stimulating"* the body's own production of required hormones, thus eliminating the many symptoms often associated with the fluctuating, or dwindling down of the body's hormone supply. At one American Cancer Society seminar in Daytona Beach, Florida, Dr. Stephen Barnes, Biochemist, University of Alabama is quoted as saying; Experimental studies involving thirty (30) rats indicated that isoflavones, naturally occurring substances found in **Soybeans and Tofu**, seemed to reduce the rate of mammary cancer in half.

Soy and its active agents are also referred to as phytoestrogens because they counter cancer-inducing estrogen (female hormone) in much the same way as the synthetic drug ***Tamoxifen*** (a synthetic hormone) does. These substances are found in regular soybeans, tofu (soybean curd), soy milk, soy flour, and miso (soybean paste), and are sold at Health Food Stores everywhere.

Suggestions for relief of Menopausal symptoms

Insomnia; Valerian capsules One or two (450 milligrams) one hour prior to bedtime.

Irritability; Caused by hormonal fluctuations. Soy products and Exercise.

Heart palpitations; See your Medical physician, and if all is well, Exercise. The heart is a muscle, Use it, or you lose it!

Lack of Energy; Cayenne capsules (goes by heat units) two on a full stomach, with 12 ounces of water. Exercise. Increased circulation results in better Oxygen utilization, and better oxygen availability improves overall energy.

Calcium loss; Request a Bone Scan if Osteoporosis is prevalent in ones family History, or if you are small framed, and of fair complexion. *If all is well, take a multiple vitamin every day for maintaining balance,*
eat lots of dark green leafy vegetables, and exercise regularly.

High Cholesterol; Supplements which have been shown to help include; Psyllium, Rice bran, and Pectin (but pectin can cause constipation if taken in excess, or without sufficient water). Also day. And remember; Exercise raises the HDL (good cholesterol), and lowers the bad, or LDL.

Weight management; Special nutritional considerations: Low fat, lower carbohydrate Diet, more fresh fruits and vegetables. Include a Chromium Supplement which helps the body to metabolize the fat, and retain a regular routine of exercise. Often its not the extra ten, or fifteen pounds one might gain, but how we carry it.

Muscle to fat composition, distribution, and often one's dress size is more important than is the slight change reflected on one's bathroom scale.

And avoid refined white sugar!

Mercury/Toxicity

by Eileen Renders N.D ~ Copyright 1998

As a Nutritional Consultant who is tuned in to symptoms as a potential signal associated with various deficiencies, imbalances and/or excess levels of one, or more of the toxic metals, an experienced Consultant (when no formal medical diagnosis has been discovered) will often recommend a Tissue Mineral Hair Analysis whenever such symptoms as nervousness, insomnia, internal shakes, and irritability are the complaint.

Suspecting an over-accumulation of one of the toxic minerals, this is exactly what is most often discovered. Often, these individuals have been prescribed potent mood altering drugs such as Zoloft, or Prozac, but these drugs can only temporarily mask the symptoms, or complaints, but do little to improve the underlying cause.

For instance;   Mercury is somewhat similar to arsenic, as it has been used medicinally. Physicians who dispensed the silvery medicine were known as quacks. This was a term that developed due to abbreviating the name quicksilver. Mercury was found in calomel lotion and was the basis for mercurial diuretics. The most well-recognized condition associated with mercury toxicity is "Hatters shakes." In years gone by, workers in hat factories were exposed to mercury in the processing of felt. You may recall the memorable character from "Alice in Wonderland" who was apparently one of those workers, the "Mad-Hatter."

Skin lightening creams were found to contain mercury. Some of these individuals developed kidney problems as a result of absorption through the organ known as the skin. Fish can also be contaminated with mercury. Accumulations from such sources readily show up in the hair. Amalgams (emollients) contain mercury and may also contribute to exposure. Mercury is used as a constituent of fungicides, algaecides and insecticides. These have contributed to mercury contamination of foods, particularly grains and cereals. Paper products and lumber contain mercury to inhibit fungus. Families have been reported to develop symptoms of mercury toxicity during the winter months from burning newspaper and building materials in their fireplaces. Mercury vapor is given off during combustion.

Mercury accumulates in tissues such as the kidney, eyes, brain, thyroid and liver. It is not uncommon to find people with hypothyroidism to have mercury toxicity. Excess mercury has been implicated in the form of cataracts. Other symptoms might include weakness of the hands, irritability, joint pain, headaches, rashes and excessive salivation. Cerebral palsy and mental retardation have been associated with mercury toxicity in children.

Modification of one's nutritional choices can help in combating the adverse effects of heavy metals. The tissue mineral analysis of zinc to mercury ratio should be at least 200:1, iron to mercury 22:1, selenium to mercury 0.8:1 and sulfur to mercury 28000:1. Zinc, selenium, iron and sulfur are helpful in combating and preventing adverse effects of mercury.

Quite often the "Cause" for one's toxicity cannot be pinpointed, however nutritional recommendations (also known as oral chelation) can bring about a return to balance in three to six months. This is done through dietary guidance, and recommendations for minerals, digestive aids, and temporary increase of opposing nutrients which assist in the removal of the excess toxic mineral.

Note: It should be noted that excess levels of one, or more of the toxic minerals quite often can cause symptoms such as nervousness, insomnia and etc. Therefore, it is understandable why many physicians prescribe medications to "Treat" the symptoms. Mercury is one of the most lethal of the toxic minerals, and over years can eventually settle in the brain, or even cause death!

Mononucleosis

by Eileen Renders N.D. Copyright 1999

Mononucleosis (Epstein Barr) is a virus which most often occurs in the young, especially teenagers, hence its nickname; "The Kissing Disease."

Symptoms associated with this disease range from malaise to sore throat, swollen glands, and may be accompanied by fever.

Confirmation of diagnosis is made through medical history, and a blood smear sample. Traditional treatment for this disease has been Steroids which may, or may not shorten the course of the illness, but which may have some effect upon glandular inflammations. However, the use of Steroids (prednisone) should be carefully weighed as the side-effects associated with the using of Steroids (cortisone) in excess can lead to;

Weakness and thinning of muscle mass, impotence, hypertension, Buffalo hump of upper back, protuberant abdomen, moon face, or purple stripes upon the body.

A large majority of Mononucleosis patients are likely to develop Strep throat, therefore a "Throat culture" is usually standard procedure, and treatable using antibiotics. The duration can be from three weeks to three months, depending upon early diagnosis, and sufficient rest.

Because fatigue is associated as a symptom with many other disorders, medical diagnosis, and treatment is not always sought immediately.

Nutritional Recommendations as Adjuvant therapy; Avoid heavy meals, as the digestive processes may be stressed, instead choose several smaller meals throughout the day. Avoid alcohol, greasy fried foods, caffeine, and an overload of processed foods.

Limit the amount of Dairy intake, but do include several fresh selections of fresh fruits, and vegetables. Consider Yogurt with Live cultures of L-Acidophilus, and foods which provide small amounts of protein which are easily digested, such as homemade chicken soup.

If possible, include rests at regular intervals throughout the day, and avoid taxing the body's energy reserves. Nourish the body with Soy protein drinks, Chinese Green tea (a good antioxidant), eggs, and plenty of dark green vegetables to insure proper chlorophyll intake.

Supplement with a good source of the Essential Fatty Acids, and provide a "Proven" Immune support supplement, such as Co-Enzyme Q-10 (60 Milligrams once daily), and support the elimination process (moving toxins out of the body) by taking 2,000 Milligrams daily of Vitamin-C at doses of 500 Milligrams four times a day. Finally, support the Liver by including 500 to 800 Milligrams a day of the Herb Blessed Thistle.

Finally, avoid Antagonist which interfere with the body's natural ability to eliminate toxins, store essential nutrients, and protect the Immune System.

Multiple Sclerosis

by Eileen Renders N.D. ~ Copyright 1998

MS is a disease noted by intermittent phases of exacerbations and remissions which are due to the progressive demyelination of the brain's white matter, and spinal cord. This disease is a major cause of disability of our adolescent population. This neurologic disorder is characterized by sporadic experiences of demyelination in various areas of the central nervous system, an occurrence which provides no warning, yet leaves in its wake, varied dysfunctional neurologic reactions. **The prognosis** for MS is somewhat unpredictable upon diagnosis, as it can often progress rapidly leading to a sudden disability, or death by early adulthood within the first six months. Yet more than 65% of MS patients lead active, and relatively comfortable lives, enjoying many long intermittent remissions.

Diagnosis: Because the initial symptoms are often so vague, or mild, recent discovery points to the fact that many MS patients often go years without being properly diagnosed. In fact, diagnosis itself requires the documentation of many neurologic attacks characterized by irritating neurologic attacks followed by lengthy periods of remissions. Magnetic Imaging will sometimes pinpoint MS legions, however, this type of testing is not foolproof. It has been found that an abnormal EEG is detected in nearly one half of MS patients, however once again, this is not an accurate test for proper diagnosing. There are other laboratory tests such as a Lumbar puncture, psychological evaluations and etc. which are useful for ruling out spinal cord compression, a foramen magnum tumor which can often mimic the symptoms of MS.

Symptoms: Depending upon the extent of destruction (including the site), including the adequacy of the bodys ability to restore the damaged, or broken down myeliniation, signs and symptoms of this disorder can vary greatly. These signs and symptoms can also be temporary, or last for weeks. Or they may present themselves with no predictable pattern, with highs and lows which change from day to day. Often, patients themselves find it difficult to describe these symptoms, another reason perhaps why MS is often difficult to diagnose. But the following symptoms are those most often described, their range of intensity however, are varied. *Visual problems (blurred), tingling or numbness, muscle weakness, including paralysis which can range from a mild muscle weakness, or tremor to a severe gait ataxia, urinary disturbances such as frequent urination, and infections, urgency and incontinence, including emotional swings, such as irritability, or euphoria to depression.*

Treatment: Physical therapy, education regarding the course of the disease, and how to manage inducers such as stress. And it is important to monitor the side effects associated with drugs used as part of therapy.

Nutritional therapy: Recommendations which are beneficial include the following: Part of the B+ complex vitamins which have been used in combination at higher doses (though this therapy **must** include incorporation of a B+ complex vitamin which contains **all** of the B vitamins, in order to eliminate the risk of inducing deficiencies in any of the other B vitamins. Doses of course, should be supervised and monitored by a skilled practitioner. *Thiamine hydrochloride* along with a multi-vitamin has been used with some success in the treatment of myasthenia gravis. Because some past research studies seemed to indicate that many types of viruses can enter the body through contaminated drinking water, invade the cells and lay dormant for a number of years, some scientists now believe that these viruses are often lethal enough to cause multiple sclerosis, and other rare nerve diseases.

Autopsy studies done on multiple sclerosis patients have shown great deficiencies of lecithin in the brain and myelin sheath which covers and protects the nerves. The minute amounts of lecithin that was found was abnormal as it contained saturated fats, rather than the necessary unsaturated fats. Based on this knowledge, a supplement of Lecithin could be extremely beneficial. The lecithin supplemented should be made of pure 100% soy in order to provide the necessary amounts of unsaturated fats (linolenic and linoleic acids). One tablespoon a day should be sufficient, and can be incorporated into a shake prepared in the blender.

Other nutrients recommended: Calcium, magnesium, vitamin D, vitamin C, and plenty of fiber derived from fresh fruits, vitamin E, trace minerals, (copper).

Lowered levels of manganese have been found in patients suffering from Downs Syndrome, Epilepsy, Schizophrenia, Parkinson disease and Multiple Sclerosis. This finding suggests a specific need for this mineral.

Some patients with Parkinson disease, Multiple sclerosis and other neuropsychiatric disorders have been reported to respond well to Cobalt therapy. This of course, would need to be discussed with one's physician.

MSM   Methylsulfonylmethane

By: Eileen Renders N. D.   Nov. 21, 2000

As always, it is of primary concern to know exactly what it is that we are putting into our body in hope of expecting some sort of therapeutic benefit. Recently MSM has found its moment of "Claim to fame", and is being used for many common disorders.

We will begin with the name itself; Methylsulfonylmethane;   methyl: according to the Webster's dictionary points to methyl as the monovalent hydrocarbon radical, normally existing only in combination, as methanol. *Monovalent meaning designating an antibody, or antigen that combines with only one specific antigen or antibody (mono always designating one).*

Sulfonyl; Meaning the divalent radical SO-2 or Sulfur. Finally "Methane"; Found in the Webster's dictionary to mean: A colorless, odorless, flammable, gaseous alkane, CH-4 present in natural gas formed by the decomposition of vegetable matter, as in marshes and mines, or produced artificially by heating

carbon monoxide and hydrogen; it is the simplest
alkane and is used as fuel, a source of carbon
black.

In short; Methylsulfonylmethane or MSM is
an organic source of sulfur, and is considered to be
one of the primary contributors in the body's
manufacture of glycosaminoglycans. Now if you
want the meaning of *gylcosaminoglycans* I suggest
that you refer to your Dictionary, Medical
dictionary, or other Nutritional and Supplement
Resource Health book, a companion that everyone
should make part of their Library collection.

Glycosaminoglycans however, are essential
constituents that comprise the bio-chemistry of the
human cartilage, the substance which cushions
and supports bone joints.

Knowing what you know now, it is somewhat
easier to make that leap from
Methylsulfonylmethane (MSM) to a supplement
for the support of joints because it not only
supports the joints (especially when it is combined
with silica and oil of anise) but reduce
inflammation. Those suffering from Arthritis,
Bursitis, and many conditions which are

diagnosed as "Itis" would benefit from supplementing the diet with MSM. Usually One (1) a day is recommended at 1,500 Milligrams, and of that, about 500 Milligrams of which is the Organic Sulfur.

Note: Many individuals taking this supplement for as little as 8 weeks claim to have found relief from pain caused by inflammation.

New Resolve

by Eileen Renders N.D. ~ Copyright 1996

We here at Renders Wellness sincerely hope that the true spirit of Christmas was able to get through all of the commercial materialism and touch your heart and spirit. If you missed the essential meaning of God's birthday because of all the hullabaloo, the aftermath often results in an overwhelming sense of depression.

If that is the case with nay of us today, it's still not too late! Visit a shut-in and bring a plateful of cheerfulness. Instead of standing in the long "Return line" at the department Store, why not take that little gift you have no use for and make it a present for the poor in your community?

Many of our senior citizens who live alone (maybe one of your neighbors) have no visitors and face a lonely existence. These are the type of gifts which will never leave us feeling "Let-down" after the holiday season is over. It is never too late to start over, to begin each day or each new week with a definite plan of doing at least one generous act for someone less fortunate than ourselves. It is this type of unselfish behavior which often lifts our own spirits, if for no other reason than to take our thoughts off of ourselves, away from what we perceive to be problems. But if you are of a deeper faith, you will be inclined to believe that any act of kindness will never go unnoticed by our creator, God. A quiet act of kindness done with no ulterior motive such as a "Reward," will become a reward in itself. This phenomenon occurs because of the positive feelings these acts seem to evoke.

On a physiological level (for those who prefer science to faith), positive emotions stimulate hormones known as endorphins. Endorphins trigger a response that has been said to actually strengthen the immune system, defeat depression and enhance an overall sense of purpose in life, which is the very key to taking better care of one's self. Perhaps that is what is meant by the hypothesis that nothing is what it seems to be!

Wrap up all that extra candy and goodies you have been gaining weight on, and take them to a nursing home resident or a shut-in neighbor. Spread good cheer and you will be overwhelmed with how that good cheer is multiplied and returned to you!

If you have, once again, overdone it, gained unwanted or unneeded pounds, don't panic! Get busy and give away those unwanted treats. Start exercising, drink more water and eat more fiber. Fiber helps to create a sense of fullness and assists one in not overeating at mealtime. Eat fruit between meals. Walk whenever time permits rather than driving. Change your life-style by instituting positive habits, and you will change your life for the better!

****

Nutrients, Concentrated (Supplements)

by Eileen Renders N.D. ~ Copyright 1999

At a time and age when many Americans are waking up to the potential risk in taking one drug after another for a lot of the common illnesses that plague many of us, we are also beginning to take a closer look at what our alternatives are: supplements and concentrated nutrients, the non-toxic remedies. These non-toxic remedies are safe and effective, when taken in proper doses and under the supervision of a practitioner qualified to make recommendations.

Renders Wellness would like to acknowledge the efforts of The Bright Side for bringing its readers continued, up-to-the-minute health information which can help to educate our community, and especially for allowing Renders Wellness to be a part of that effort in providing this Health column since 1995. Health Maintenance/Disease Prevention can lengthen not only one's life span, but the very quality of life itself while helping to maintain a chronic disorder.

Often we are asked to review a particular product, and provide a professional opinion regarding same. The product in question is known as OPC-3. It is a formula which combines grape seed extract (which helps us to maintain proper internal ph), Red wine extract (which has been shown by several studies in France to reduce high lipid levels in the blood and bioflavonoids which lessen the allergy response to harmless substances, and protect the arteries from damage caused by free-radicals.

OPC-3 (along with Aloe) has recently received recognition from its many users for its benefit in clearing up several skin problems such as eczema. Because the skin is the body's largest organ, it has long be vulnerable to eruptions which are part of the body's defense mechanism for throwing off toxins. Grape seed extract (which is part of the OPC-3 formulation) has been shown to contain strong anti-viral, and anti-bacterial properties.

This particular combination of nutrients may also bestow other benefits such as; Assist in preventing Strokes by inhibiting excess accumulation of fibrin (clotting factor), and also by lowering serum cholesterol levels. These seem to be products that I would recommend.

Note: On an individual basis, Grape Seed Extract wins hands down for its potency and effectiveness as a non-toxic antioxidant!

Nutritional therapy

by   Eileen Renders N.D. Copyright 1999

Because I was fortunate enough to be led, and early on in my Practice, sensed the real need for an emphasis on specific nutrients to address deficiencies of long duration, many specific nutrients were recommended to the hundreds of Clients who passed through our doors, each meant to address a specific ailment, without giving-in to the ingesting of yet another drug that was meant to suppress the symptoms associated with the taking of the "First" drug.

We worked through the Atlantic City Medical Center's HIV Consortium, a program funded by The Ryan White Funding as set up by the N.I.H. (National Institutes of Health), and helped the HIV/AIDS through ; *Nutritional support (teaching them what were Antagonists, and what therefore, to avoid), Guided Imagery (to reduce, and manage Stress), and Herbal recommendations (using only Researched, and "Proven" herbs) to boost the Immune System.*

We work with Cancer patients who are undergoing Chemotherapy, and knowing how the toxic drugs used to kill cancer do not differentiate between cancer cells, or healthy cells, we moved to "over-compensate" with specific nutrients which would assist the body to continue to build new healthy cells, even in the presence of Chemo drugs. We have seen children die not from recurrent cancers, but from the aggressive forms of treatment which led to Liver failure. We are not saying that the Chemotherapy was not indicated, but we are saying that; *Nutritional therapy, detoxification, and Immune enhancement* are the only safe, and often effective forms of Adjuvant therapies available which make good sense.

Nutrition has traditionally been associated with Athletes who wish to make use of concentrated nutrients, or Amino Acids for the purpose of burning fat, building muscle, or increasing stamina, and Dietitians for the most part are known for their ability to Teach us how to eat more nutritiously, but this is not what Nutritional therapy is all about.

Concentrated nutrients are therapeutic when one has the knowledge, and experience to

recommend those which are safe, and can ;
Lower blood lipid cholesterol levels, reduce
inflammation, or work much like a Pro-biotic, or
Analgesic.

Too, we have all recognized the fact that we
are not all "Created equal", but are subject to our
unique, and often identifiable genetic weaknesses.

All of which translates to mean that the RDA, or
Recommended Daily Allotments which have been
determined for us by the State Health Dept.
Guidelines are Minimal daily allotments.
Whenever one has a deficiency of long duration,
or a genetic weakness which requires "more" of a
specific nutrient in order to assist one's body to
operate on a normal level, or to over-compensate
for the toxic effects which are associated with
Chemotherapy, are all circumstances wherein
Nutritional therapy can work to help the body gain
strength and balance, and to eliminate the
possibility of further compromising one's Immune
System.

This Article is written for all who practice
Health, yet are not aware of the benefits associated
with Nutritional therapy, those who instinctively

realize that they want "more" than the traditional therapy they are receiving, and for those Practitioners who have requested an explanation regarding "What it is?"

Note: We are very proud to be associated with, and may be the first Nutritional Practice to coin the term "Nutritional therapy!"

Obesity ~ Appetite ~ Overeating ~
By: Eileen Renders N. D.
Copyright 1999

If food ingested becomes energy (especially complex carbohydrates), it is easy to understand how weight management has much to do with the theory; *energy (*calories*)* consumed should not be more than calories (*energy)* spent in a day. And we have read and learned much about our *Metabolism,* and the meaning of thermogenesis. In fact, it is rather common knowledge today, that in order to *reduce one's total weight,* it is often necessary to both reduce one's caloric intake, while at the same time, increasing one's activity. That is sort of like putting out more than one is taking in.

However, knowing that one has a specific problem does not help one manage that problem, that is;   Without further knowledge!   For instance;   Many individuals who attempt to do just that, reduce their caloric intake while increasing their activity, often complain of the increased appetite that follows a good workout!

The result is often overeating, rather than selective, or restrictive eating!

So to what can we attribute this increased hunger? And how can we begin to attempt to manage this increased hunger? One theory is that a low blood glucose concentration, or impaired glucose utilization is responsible for triggering the "Hunger" response. Another factor involved in metabolism is heat. Often one's body temperature is associated with metabolism. Perhaps that is why those with a condition known as hyperthyroidism are always cold, able to eat whatever they please, and never gain a pound. During exercise (or shivering), body heat rises, but during sleep heat production and the metabolic rate drops to about 10% below the BMR, or Basil Metabolism Rate.

In fever, the appetite often decreases, and it is the release of chemicals from the *hypothalamus,* known as *pyrogen's* which are in part, responsible for maintaining body temperature (such as utilizing heat created during exercise, by increasing metabolism temporarily).

*It is also believed that the hypothalamus which regulates the body's heat and assists in regulating metabolism, **is also involved in regulating the appetite!***

Blood glucose concentration (also involved in appetite) is associated with the pancreas. Without elaborating too much, glycolysis is the breakdown of glucose in order to provide cells with energy. Gluconeogenesis however, is the formation of "new glucose" which is comprised of proteins, or the glycerol of fats, and not from carbohydrates. The complex mechanism which maintains homeostasis of blood sugar concentration is made possible by hormonal and neural devices, in fact, five endocrine glands; Islands of Langerhans, anterior, pituitary gland, adrenal cortex, adrenal medulla, and thyroid glands, and at least eight hormones secreted by those glands function as primary parts to the homeostatic mechanism of blood sugar mechanism, and is involved with reactions by the appetite control center!

Now there is no need to study, memorize, or attempt to decipher the above information with regard to understanding one's metabolic rate, body weight, or appetite control center, however the point of this article is to open up the door to understanding exactly "How important" it is to one's health, and weight management goals, that all internal organs are functioning optimally and harmoniously.

Nutrients are relative to homeostasis as much as internal organs and glands optimum performance are relative to one's optimum state of well being, or health.

****

Olive Leaf Extract

By: Eileen Renders

The Olive tree was first recorded centuries
ago, and is mentioned quite frequently in the
Bible. Used mostly in the kitchen today because of
its unique ability for lowering the LDL (or bad
cholesterol) that shows up in our blood, the Olive
leaf in concentrated forms becomes an Extract,
and offers other medicinal benefits, and has been
studied for years.

The University of Texas Health Science
Center in Dallas reports that over two million
people across the entire United States are leaving
hospitals with a "Hospital acquired" infection
caused by nosocomial exposure. And the Center
relates that as many as 22,000 Americans will
succumb to their infections. The reason for this
alarming fact is because "The life-saving
technology that once saved lives, sets them up for
infection." At least that is what Robert Haley,
M.D., and head of the Epidemiology and
Preventive Medicine Unit at the University of
Texas Health Science Center has said.

Moreover, antibiotic-resistant organisms are a real potential resulting from any infection, regardless of its cause. Dr. Haley further states that as the cost of an antibiotic comes down, our resistance to its (the antibiotic) effectiveness goes up. Not so surprising then, should it be to us, after forty years of "Treating patients" for various major (or minor) problems with antibiotics, that these bacteria have mutated themselves, building up strong defenses against what was once, a powerful "Miracle" drug.

While antibiotics never really were effective against a virus anyway, we now must protect ourselves against infections, or the need for the use of antibiotics. But how?

1.- Insure that our nutritional intake is adequate.
2.- Manage stress effectively, as it robs us of our life giving nutrients. 3.- Consistently manage stress through daily practices of one, or more of the following; Exercise, prayer, Guided Imagery, or Meditation. 4.- Employ the super antioxidants in with our supplemental regime, antioxidants such as; Selenium, Beta carotene, Zinc, CO-Enzyme-Q-10 (a bioflavonoid.) 5.- Avoid

constipation (a source of toxins), as it is a high associative symptom often linked to colorectal cancer. 6.- Enhance the Immune System through a daily supplement of vitamin-C (which also helps to rid the body of toxins.)

Finally, educate yourself, and protect your family through incorporating the use of the many effective natural antibiotics available to us today. Olive Leaf Extract might very well be considered among that list.

Olive Leaf Extract was proven, through various Research Studies at Northwestern University Medical School by Gary A. Noskin, M.D., Assistant Professor of Medicine reported that Olive Leaf Extract (in vitro) was an effective treatment against "Aspergillus prasiticus", and various other strains of lactic acid bacteria. Other Studies showing some of Olive Leaf's benefits included the Division of Biologics, PHLS Centre for Applied Microbiology and Research in Porton Down, Salisbury, Wilts, United Kingdom, and in other Studies conducted in Italy by several other Ph.D.'s

Note: It is import to also be advised that any treatment should only e undertaken under the guidance and advisement of a skilled practitioner. Dosage, frequency and length of therapy can counteract any of the possible benefits, and other considerations for recommendations include; Disorder, age, weight, and etc.

In conclusion, Olive Leaf Extract may well be effective in the short term treatment of such conditions as Chronic Fatigue where Epstein-Barr has been diagnosed.

****

ORGANIC FLAX OIL

Copyright 1998

By: Eileen Renders N. D.

Biochemists who evaluate various forms of the Omega 3, Omega 6, *Essential Fatty Acids,* the unsaturated fats, also known as linoleic and linolenic acids, conduct their Evaluations by considering each oils individual molecular structure, along with the length of their "Bonding chains." According to many Experts, and one in particular (Dr. Johanna Budwig of Europe, who was nominated seven times for her the Nobel Prize Award, because of her work in the study of fats), one stands alone, above all the rest. *The Essential Fatty acids source which holds the title as being "The strongest, purest form of the Essential Fatty Acids, and that is Organic Flax oil."*

Because it is a cold pressed oil, it must be kept refrigerated, and never heated, or it could become oxidized, and turn rancid.. They Essential Fatty Acids (linolenic and linoleic acids) are referred to as "Essential" because while they are essential for good nutrition, the body has not the ability to manufacture them, therefore, they must be obtained through nutritional sources.

Here is a partial list of some of the many health benefits derived from supplementing one's diet with one (1) tablespoonful daily, of organic flax oil:

~ Reduces the LDL, or "Bad-   cholesterol"

~ Raises the HDL, or "Good" cholesterol"

~ It reduces the amount of Histamine that is released by the body in response to allergens.

~ It reduces inflammation

~ Stimulates the production of neurotransmitters that are necessary for the brain in order to send messages to various parts of the body.

~ Helps to clean the walls of the arteries, and prevent Arteriosclerosis.

~ It works in conjunction with other nutrients in preserving the strength, and health of the bones joints.

~ An absolute requirement for optimum health of the Skin, Nails and Hair.

~   It stimulates a response within the body
      which is very similar as that
      response that occurs between plants and
      Sunlight, known as "Photosynthesis."

EXERCISE

By: Eileen Renders N. D.

For individuals who may want to exercise regularly, but are not sufficiently motivated, please consider the following Health benefits which are benefits of a regular Exercise routine:

~   Increases bone density, especially Walking, and "weight-bearing" exercises.

~   Stimulates the manufacture of hormones, which are required in order to optimally carry out normal internal processes.

~   It is a "Natural Stress Reliever", as it is known to release hormones (Endorphins, in particular) which reduce the Stress level.

~   It strengthens the Heart, which is a muscle (*Use It, Or Lose It!),* and helps to reduce the risk for Heart disease.

~   Lowers cholesterol (total blood lipid levels.)

~   Assists in helping to maintain proper weight, and management of the same.

~   Induces better sleep patterns.

~   Increases Metabolism.

~   Stimulates internal organs to perform better;

kidneys, bowels, heart, and etc. thereby reducing chances of constipation, water retention, or heart disease!

~ Muscle weighs more than fat, and allows for a higher caloric intake.

~ Enhances circulation, oxygen utilization, thereby raising energy levels.

****

OSTEOARTHRITIS

By: Eileen Renders N. D.

Osteoarthritis is a degenerative bone disease which is the most common form of bone disorder effecting the elderly. Its onset can occur anywhere between the ages of 40 and 60, and is a disorder which is identified by loss of articular (a point of contact between two joints) cartilage along with new bone formation which hinders proper movement. **Causes;** There are two types of Osteoarthritis, Primary and Secondary. Primary Osteoarthritis is a normal part of the aging process and is greatly influenced by the following; Chemical, genetic, mechanical and/or metabolic factors. Secondary Osteoarthritis usually occurs after other events; Congenital deformity, obesity or trauma. **Symptoms;** The commonest symptom which accurately describes Osteoarthritis is a deep, unrelenting pain which originates from deep within a specific joint. It can be triggered by a weight bearing exercise (especially those involving a particular afflicted area), changes in the weather, or occupational stress. **Diagnosis;** A physical examination can rule out an inflammatory joint disease, and X-rays of the affected area can confirm diagnosis. Bony deposits and joint deformities will confirm diagnosis.

Traditional medical treatment; Depending upon the affected area and/or the severity of the problem, medical treatment can vary. For instance; If the hip is the affected area, and walking becomes too painful, surgery to remove and replace the deformed bone may be suggested.

If the Osteoarthritis is limited to the hand joints (Osteoarthritis is not a systemic disease ~ meaning that it usually only affects specific areas), hot soaks may be helpful. For pain, analgesics such as aspirin are recommended, and in severe cases, steroid injections a couple of times a year has often been the treatment.

Note: The first signs of Osteoarthritis are very meek, and are often explained as "Morning stiffness", but as the disease advances, the pain of motion in the affected area is aggravated by prolonged use, and is only lessened through rest. There is usually no inflammation.

Rheumatoid arthritis on the other hand, is a chronic inflammatory condition that affects the entire body, and most specifically the synovial membranes of the joints. It is referred to as an "Auto immune" disease because the body's immune system attacks its own body. In rheumatoid arthritis, it is the hands, wrists, ankle and feet (sometimes knees) that are most affected. Fever, fatigue and stiffness are the first complaints of this disorder, however without intervention there soon will be swollen joints in a few weeks making normal range of movement painful.

Causes;   What triggers this autoimmune disorder is largely unknown, yet many studies seem to point toward genetic predisposition toward rheumatoid arthritis. This explanation however, does not rule out other contributing factors such as environmental, and/or nutritional.

Nutritional and herbal considerations;

~   Avoid highly processed foods

~   Limit caffeine, sugar and alcohol

~   Institute regular exercise program

~   Water intake of quart and a half

~   Daily multiple vitamin

Glucosamine chondroitin

~   topical cream containing *Capsicum frutescence,* Cayenne or Salicylic Acid~ Essential Fatty Acids (*preferably one tablespoonful of organic Flax oil daily)*

~   Tumeric ~ Two/Three capsules daily helps to reduce inflammation and therefore, reduce pain. Glucosamine Chondroitin with MSM is also useful..

****

PHOSPHOROUS

by: Eileen Renders N. D. ~   Copyright Mar, 2001

An essential mineral, phosphorous is the second most abundantly found mineral in the body .It is present in every cell and is involved in nearly every chemical reaction within the body. In fact, one part phosphorous to every 2.5 parts of Calcium helps to maintain healthy bones. *This required balance is upset in the presence of refined white sugar.* Phosphorous is also beneficial in assisting the body to manufacture phospholipids, such as lecithin, which aid the body in metabolizing and transporting fats.

This mineral is also intricately involved in the synthesis of deoxyribonucleic acid (DNA), the coding which carries the messages for cell replication and life, and ribonucleic acid (RNA). Also, it has been utilized successfully to speed up the healing process of bone fractures and for the treatment of Osteoporosis. Some research suggests that phosphorous may provide some protection against cancer. Deficiencies in phosphorous include metabolic disturbances, bone degeneration, changes in normal weight patterns, and appetite and/or memory impairment. There is no known toxicity associated with phosphorous intake. The RDA (Recommended Daily Allowance) for phosphorous is from 800 to 1,600 micrograms, depending upon variable factors such as sex, and age. If the body's Calcium is too high, additional phosphorous can be taken to bring about a return of balance. Natural sources of phosphorous include;   Meat, fish, whole grains, nuts, milk and dairy products, sesame seeds, and Brewer's yeast.

Note: The above information and more can be found in; FOOD ADDITIVES, NUTRIENTS AND SUPPLEMENTS A TO Z ~

By Eileen Renders N. D.

****

PMS ~ Premenstrual Syndrome

by: Eileen Renders N. D.

Copyright: September, 2000

A condition which now effects many women between the ages of 20 and 40 years of age, PMS (Pre Menstrual Syndrome) can include many of the following symptoms;   Tenderness felt in the breasts, headache, irritability, depression bloating, backache, diminished sex drive, fatigue, tension, and swelling of the ankles and fingers.

Symptoms which seem to appear anywhere from between 7 to 14 days prior to the onset of the menses, these symptoms can become quite severe for many women, yet there seems to be little done to date through clinical studies. One common denominator which appears to be prevalent between women suffering with PMS, yet absent in women without PMS symptoms as Dr. Michael T. Murray N. D. points out for us is that there exists a pattern of elevated plasma Estrogen along with a decrease of plasma Progesterone levels in these women about 5 to 10 days prior to menstruation.

Doctor David Watts makes another interesting point in relating to us how Estrogen is closely related with copper levels, and as one rises, so too, does the other. Zinc is associated with progesterone levels, and the levels of these two is said to move in tandem. Doctor Watts further states that many women taking oral contraceptives have an elevated level of copper. In fact, many gynecologists believe that it is the elevated copper absorption which prevents conception.

It is common to find women who suffer PMS to have elevated tissue copper levels. Copper levels also affect the menstrual flow; high tissue copper levels, potential for prolonged and/or heavy menstrual flow.

Recommendations for relieving symptoms associated with PMS; Vitamin B-6, Zinc, Vitamin -C, Vitamin-E, and the herb Chasteberry.

****

Rhubarb

by Eileen Renders N.D.   Copyright 1999

Native to China, Siberia and India, rhubarb is widely cultivated in many geographic areas. Sturdy perennials which commonly grow to nearly 10 feet high, they are known for their huge, strong leaves. There are the garden varieties which are utilized for their edible stalks which is abundant in several minerals, including calcium, potassium, and phosphorus. And then there is the Chinese rhubarb which is said to more utilized for its medicinal value.

In China, rhubarb juice and tea is employed in the treatment of cancer with documented success. The initial issue of Pharmacology (Vol. 20) printed that two of rhubarb's constituents which are said to have a laxative effect (rhein and emodin) were shown in laboratory tests to inhibit mammary tumors in mice by as much as 75%. And the Journal of Ethno pharmacology printed in one 1984 issue how those same two substances (rhein and emodin) inhibited the growth of malignant melanoma when given at a dose of 50 milligrams per kilogram of body weight each day.

And a rhubarb root liquid solution was given in daily oral doses to rabbits which were both normal and hyperlipidemic (high lipid blood levels.) Rabbits that had begun the experiment with elevated cholesterol and tryglyceride levels experienced impressive decreases in these levels, and it has been suggested that rhubarb may be beneficial for maintaining a healthy lipid level, and should be included at the end of a big meal, especially those which are high in fat.

Besides its anti-tumor benefit, rhubarb is also thought to be effective in relieving the itch often associated with psoriasis. Other claims have been that rhubarb lessens the pain which often accompanies Arthritis.

In Shanghai in the 1980's, Chinese rhubarb was used in a Study that included nearly 1000 individuals who experienced upper digestive tract bleeding (more than 50% were duodenal ulcers that were complicated by hemorrhaging), and were treated with either rhubarb powder, tablets, or syrup. They were administered 1 teaspoon three times a day until the bleeding ceased, averaging about two days with most. A 97%

success rate was realized.

Depending upon the dose, rhubarb can correct constipation, or halt diarrhea.

Note: Rhubarb is low in calories and fat, a fair source of fiber, but because it is tart, it can be mixed with fruit to become more palatable.

The Calcium available in rhubarb is generally not able to be utilized by the body because it also contains oxalic acid. Oxalic acid binds to the calcium, therefore making it difficult to utilize, or store.

Best way to eat; Cook, strain and mix with honey.

Scleroderma ~ Nutrients & Herbs

by; Eileen Renders N. D. Copyright 2000

Scleroderma ~ Reticular tissue forms the framework for the Spleen, lymph nodes and bone marrow.

Collagen ~ "Hyaluronidase" is an enzyme which gives collagen its viscous quality. It is stretchable, loose, ordinary connective tissue, an elastic glue. Of the half dozen or so kinds of cells present, **fibroblasts** are the most common variety, and **macrophages** are second.   Connective tissue is formed from protein.

Scleroderma is an autoimmune disease which is fast becoming a common disorder with previously unknown etiologies (cause.)   In autoimmune disease, auto antibodies (AABs) are produced by B Lymphocytes and they attack normal cells that have a "Self" antigen, or auto antigen (AAG).   This process causes inflammation and destruction of the tissue.

Nutritional recommendations ~ Initially, a Tissue Mineral Hair Analysis is strongly recommended for the purpose of correcting nutritional deficiencies, and balancing of other excess (often toxic) minerals such as Lead, Mercury, Aluminum often a contributing factor for faulty Immune responses.

The next process with a goal in mind for optimum management of a chronic disorder is to begin a detoxification process which would include educational information regarding; Dietary habits, avoidance of potential antagonists (substances which interfere with normal internal functioning), and finally;   The third step would be recommendations for nutrients and at least one (1) proven safe and effective herb to be taken at proper dosage for short term intervals.   Short term therapeutic doses work best therapeutically as they eliminate the possibility of declining beneficial effects due to what is known as the tolerance factor.   Sulfur such as found in Garlic is beneficial to the health of the tissue, as is Silica which is found in the herb Horsetail.   And now MSM Methylsulfonylmethane.   See more or MSM under that heading.

EFA ~ Essential fatty acids are also beneficial.

Caution: There are other nutrients (concentrated forms are therapeutic) and/or herbs which complete the above partial protocol, and doses and length of duration should always be supervised by a professional. Contraindications must also be a consideration.

Selenium

by Eileen Renders N. D.

An essential mineral, Selenium was first noticed because of its potential for toxicity, and later in the 18th century for its beneficial uses in industries such as xerographic and photocopying. Interest in its ability to provide beneficial effects in humans came about only after the selenium compound named "Factor 3." Factor 3 was shown after much clinical research to provide animals with protection caused from fatty infiltration of the liver. In 1957 researchers at the National Institutes of Health discovered that there was a definite association between a selenium deficiency and abnormalities in laboratory animals. When selenium supplementation showed reversal of some specific abnormalities, that led to further research. It was found that selenium was involved with certain enzymes relative to cellular oxidation. About that time, the generalization was that selenium was also involved in human nutrition as well. Selenium deficiencies are rare today and is found in many staple foods.

At one time however, a disease known as Keshan disease (cardiomyopathy effecting mostly children) was found in children and young women living in China in areas where the soil was poor in selenium content. Selenium has been found in low levels in individuals with cataracts, as well as those with certain types of iron deficiencies. High levels of free radical production and/or a lowered ability to inhibit the production of these free radicals is thought by some experts to speed up the aging process. Other studies have indicated that selenium provides protection on mammary tumor formation and reduced tumor growth rates in animals. Low levels of selenium, and vitamin-E, show a direct correlation to certain types of cancer; Gastrointestinal, lung and skin. There are several traceable factors which contribute to a selenium deficiency, such as; Excessive levels of Sulfur (a mineral which protects the body from Selenium toxicity), silver, arsenic, cadmium, and mercury. Still, when ratios between selenium and Zinc or Copper are out of balance, an antagonistic effect to selenium is imposed.

As stated earlier on however, selenium was known for its toxicity long before it was discovered for its antioxidant benefits. Selenium toxicity has been linked to such industries as; Ore extraction, mining, including zinc, lead, pyrite roasting, and the producing of lime and cement. Symptoms of selenium toxicity are described as; Eye irritation, nose, throat, burning sensation of nostrils, sneezing, coughing, congestion , dizziness, dyspnea, headaches and edema. Symptoms associated with high supplementation of selenium might include any or all of the following;   Hair loss, nausea, vomiting, skin depigmentation, irritability and peripheral neuropathy. **Selenium food sources include;** Tuna, herring, Brewer's yeast, wheat germ and bran, whole grains and sesame seeds. **Daily guidelines:** Infants 0.01-0.06 milligrams, children; 0.02-0.2 milligrams, adults 0.05-0.2 milligrams.

ALLERGIES AND SINUSITIS

By: Eileen Renders N. D.

Copyright July, 2001

Each year, more and more individuals are complaining of Seasonal allergies from Pollen, Ragweed, dust and/or various types of foods. These allergies take on new meaning however, as many of these individuals now complain that their response to these allergens far surpass the traditional "Seasonal" type of allergies. And a more serious problem now exists because often times, one of the symptoms associated with a specific type of response to allergens (post nasal drip) frequently leads to Sinus infections.

Traditional treatment through the use of Antibiotics is often effective, but when the hyper-sensitive individual is left with a yeast infection or gastrointestinal problems due to the frequent use of antibiotics, those individuals now have yet another serious problem to deal with. Therefore, what seems to be lacking here in traditional treatment of Allergies is how to manage the symptoms, without having to resort to an antibiotic each time an individual with Sinus problems (post nasal drip) begins to experience a sore throat, which can be quite often!

As an N. D. Doctor of Naturopathy, it is my belief that *prevention* and/or *management* of these common disorder is crucial. Continuous ingestion of antibiotics leaves it mark by reducing one's tolerance or ability to respond to these antibiotics, AND while antibiotics DO kill bacteria, they also distinguish the good bacteria, or intestinal flora that defends the body against many species of bacteria.

After using any antibiotic it is imperative to replenish that intestinal flora with a high potency pro-biotic containing L-Acidophilus, Lactobacillus casel, Lactobacillus plantarum and etc.

With allergies which cause excess mucus, it is best to avoid meat and dairy products for awhile. Replace with Rice, Goat or Soy milk. Protein can be found in Rice and Beans, Rice and Corn (only in combination), chicken, fish and protein drinks. Meat and Dairy products have been shown to cause many of the following symptoms in hyper-sensitive individuals;   Hives,

Sinusitis, heart disorders, excess mucus, hormonal imbalances, diarrhea, edema, dermatitis, acne, impaired digestion, constipation, bloating, colic and other symptoms as well.

Individuals with food allergies report good results through the use of; Green tea, and non-dairy yogurts.

With catarrh (excess mucus), a combination of Echinacea and Golden Seal seems to reduced symptoms, as well as Bioflavonoids along with Vitamin-C a couple of times a day. At first sign of a sore throat, implement an intervention of Garlic oil capsules in order to prevent a Sinus infection. And drink plenty of water to flush out toxins!

****

Sodium, Potassium

by Eileen Renders N. D.

Copyright August, 2000

Blood levels of Minerals are indicative of the type of internal communication going on internally, and specific to one's biochemical profile. However, a routine blood test is not accurate at pinpointing people who may, or may not be, sodium sensitive (or insensitive). A pattern which can contribute to high blood pressure. On the contrary, many individuals who suffer from hypertension due to sodium sensitivity (or essential hypertension) will show no clues to this type of high blood pressure, or imbalances at all within the electrolytes upon examination.

However, there exists a reliable screening procedure for showing a link, or tendency in certain individuals for the onset of hypertension relative to sodium sensitivity. That test is known as a TMA, or Tissue Mineral Analysis.

A ratio of 2.4:1. is generally considered the norm, or ideal relationship between Sodium and Potassium. While high tissue levels of sodium and potassium relative to calcium and magnesium

197

reflect fast adrenal activity, this activity is also often associated with a high level stress response, and common in *fast metabolizers*. This type of individual is more prone to such disorders as; Anxiety, cardiovascular disease, hypertension and hyperthyroidism. Also, high levels of sodium and potassium are associated with stress reactions and/or the onset of an inflammatory problem.

On the other hand, low levels of sodium and potassium (especially sodium) relative to calcium and magnesium is a mineral profile which often reflects the *slow metabolizer,* and is therefore, commonly found in such conditions as; Adrenal exhaustion, chronic fatigue, depression, hypoglycemia and hypothyroidism. In fact, these minerals (sodium and potassium relative to other minerals such as calcium and magnesium, phosphorus and iron) provide the practitioner with the biochemistry information which can point to Adrenal activity, and/or the ability to predict which individuals may be vulnerable to sodium sensitivity and a relationship to high blood pressure.

Renders Wellness can provide a TMA which

analyzes for 36 essential nutrients, including six toxic metals such as;   Mercury Aluminum, Lead, Arsenic & etc.

****

SOY

By: Eileen Renders N. D.

Copyright 1996

SOY...Little word, but definitely not the last word on the known benefits and experiments surrounding soy. But, separate fact from the hype may require concentrating our attention on what we know to be true.

Soybeans (Glycine or Soja max). Unlike most beans which originate from the genus "Phaseoulous," the soybean is distinctive right from the start. They are firm, round and rather bland tasting. For the true vegetarian, soy offers, among other nutrients, a valuable source of protein.

Phyto chemicals (meaning its origin is from plant life) contain certain compounds which protect us from cancer (such as anti-carcinogens), or which can stimulate and/or balance the production of other natural occurring hormones within the body. Initial studies now lead present day researches to believe that soy may even inhibit replication and growth of certain diseases, such as cancer and HIV. Among Institutions and/or Organizations studying Soy is the National Cancer Institute.

In certain types of cancer, such as breast cancer, soy, it appears, has the ability of inhabiting certain "Receptor sites" which might otherwise become invaded and inhabited by cancer cell formations. It appears that the female hormone estrogen is responsible for creating these inviting little "Receptor areas;" it is the chemical known as "Indoles" which is found in certain foods, such as soy, which takes up these receptor sites making the opportunity for certain types of cancers unlikely.

While such studies have not totally confirmed these findings, there is strong suggestion that adding a bit of tofu or tempa to your diet can be most beneficial. If the receptor site theory proves true, then soy may also be beneficial to HIV patients, as soy may also protect against replication of HIV Studies of Japanese men found that there is a direct link between tofu consumption and lower rates of prostate cancer. Soy seems to show that it can inhibit the growth of these cancer cells in laboratory cultures.

Other statements regarding the benefits of soy

are endless. It has been said that soy has the ability to assist the body in lowering LDL cholesterol readings for certain individuals and that soybeans' peptides can even give the immune system a boost! Still other researchers in Japan believe that these compound, referred to as phytoestrogens, can also help alleviate the annoying symptoms often associated with menopause.

As you might expect, soy is much easier on the filtering systems (the kidneys) than protein derived from animals, and therefore often recommended with individuals suffering from kidney damage.

Tofu, which is derived from the soybean, is rather bland. But, adding a low sodium soy sauce along with fresh vegetables and seasonings can produce a "Healthy burger" substitute. Using your imagination, tofu can become a substitute ingredient for eggs or butter and can even become party of your next "Cheesecake!"
Soy, "Its wazzup!"

****

"How Sweet It Is", A Matter of Taste

By: Eileen Renders N. D.   Copyright 1996

"How Sweet It Is" was a phrase most often associated with the late comedian Jackie Gleason, one of my television favorites. And after Jackie, another association and favorite treat used in America today, is sugar!

There is glucose, sucrose, fructose, lactose, maltose, and starch. While most of us are aware that sugar is found in high content candy, ice cream, pastries, jams and heavy syrups, many may be unaware that it can also be found in high content in such foods as breakfast cereals, baby foods, salad dressings, soups and even in yogurt and granola bars.

While most of us are aware of the link between simple carbohydrates and obesity, many researchers suspect there is a definite connection between these same simple carbohydrates (refined white sugar) and heart disease and diabetes, though there is no proven certainty published at this time.

Over consumption of starch and sweet foods in the diet can often result in a nutritional deficiency as they are lacking in essential nutrients, especially in one of the more needed vitamins, such as the B vitamins, and can, therefore, often perpetuate such symptoms as heartburn, indigestion or nausea. Other research continues as to whether or not refined carbohydrates contribute to such disorders as high blood pressure, anemia, kidney disease and cancer.

On a more positive note, thousands of years ago, Egyptians packed serious wounds with honey and other sweet substances. These treatments fell into disuse, particularly after the discovery of antibiotics. Yet in some parts of Europe, there are physicians who still use sugar to treat bedsores. It appears to be effective, in that it dehydrates the area being treated of infectious bacteria. It is an inexpensive treatment which doctors have used, because it seems to heal wounds rather quickly. SUGGESTION: While refined white sugar may or may not contribute to the onset of disease, our recommendation is to use a substitute which can be easily assimilated by the body and efficiently utilized. One that is full of valuable nutrients (B vitamins) is rice malt syrup or granules, which can be purchased at your local health food store. In baking, consider replacing refined white sugar with unsweetened, concentrated frozen white grape juice.

Stevia (herb) can be purchased at your local Health Food Store as well as Date Sugar, nutritious Barley malt granules (100 times sweeter than refined white sugar), and other healthier replacements.

Note: In 2001 the new and improved Stevia has added the following ingredients;

Inulin ~ A type of sugar derived from plants. Inulin is also used medicinally by injection for determining kidney function, and is often found in bread for diabetics.

Chromium ~ (from Chromium Chelavite (Trademark) Chromium has long been found to Be involved in the breakdown of sugar in metabolism, but is often deficient in our diets due to many geographic soil deficiencies!

****

For The Family Pet

by Eileen Renders N. D.   Copyright 1997

While puppies and cats have long become an
extra family member, we also recognize their
value in hundreds of Nursing and Convalescent
Homes across the United States. Their visits to
such facilities it has been noted, have significantly
lifted the moods and spirits of many shut-in's,
alleviated depression in some and even lowered
blood pressure readings of others.

Therefore, we can easily understand the
concern of such pet owners when their "Extra"
family members is not feeling well. In this close
relationship between the family pet and the owner,
the responsibility of taking care of the pet's needs
can often put a dent into the family budget.
Remembering that should your pet become ill or
exhibit serious symptoms such as fever, loss of
appetite, noticeable weight loss or other symptoms
which may require the expertise of a Veterinarian,
we hope that you do not hesitate to do so.

For minor problems which might save you an
unnecessary trip to the Vet along with the added
cost of pet prescriptions, you may want to

consider a few of the following;

- Black Walnut Extract: Kills and expels worms
- Cascara Sagrada: Relieves constipation, improves digestion
- Cornsilk: Soothes inflammation of the kidney-bladder
- Echinacea: Boosts the immune response and helps to keep your pet healthy
- Red Raspberry: Strengthens the uterus, helpful in labor prior to delivery
- Tea Tree Oil: Antifungal, add to bath water regularly to kill fleas
- Valerian Extract: Calming helpful when given prior to a nail clipping or grooming
- Vitamin E: 400 I. U., (the heart and circulation vitamin)
- Yellow Dock: Made into a tea and used to swab the ears may prevent ear mites
- Zinc: 25 mg. Can encourage a healthy coat growth, hormones and speed healing

Tick Season

By: Eileen Renders N. D.   Copyright 1997

We waited a long time to once again get out of doors and enjoy some of those good old back yard barbecues. The sun is shining, the pollen's finally down and the flowers are blooming, all of which often overwhelm our senses with a false sense of security! I don't want to spoil your picnic, but don't allow yourself to be lulled into complacency, especially out there under the shade trees or walking in the grass.

Take precautions to prevent a deer tick bite. Protect yourself and your children by wearing socks and shoes, as opposed to sandals. Wear, white as often as possible to make it easier to detect ticks on you. Buy a repellent and lightly spray your clothes before putting them on. This will protect you and minimize any toxins from being absorbed through skin (especially important for children).

Soon after returning back inside, immediately check one another's backs, necks and other parts of your body for ticks. If alone, take a quick shower to rinse off any ticks which may not yet have bitten the skin.

Check with your local garden center or pet supply store and pick up a bag of tick repellent. Studies have shown that when this tick repellent is mixed with water in an aerosol spray vessel, and sprayed lightly around your back yard, it can effectively prevent ticks from multiplying and lurking, waiting for a host. However, since this chemical is toxic, directions are critical. It should not be sprayed where pets or animals feed, or near flower or vegetable gardens.

Be aware of the symptoms and signs which might indicate that one has unknowingly been bitten. One of the first signs is a rash, which appears as a circle surrounding that spot where on has been injected with the deer tick's poison. Other signs include fatigue, fever, aches and pains described as the type which initiate at the deepest level, or in the bone.

As with any other disorder or disease, time is of the essence. The sooner one has been examined, tested and diagnosed, the quicker one can begin treatment. If you have been bitten, tape the tick to an index card and mail it off for testing to find out whether or not the tick is infected with Lyme Disease. Mail to: Joint Tick Project, 123 Huntington Street, New Haven Connecticut, 06504. There is no charge for this service.

Don't wait until the results are returned, as they could take as long as several weeks. Most physicians will not begin a lot of testing; they will opt to initiate treatment at once through prescribed several weeks of antibiotics. The longer the disease is allowed to remain in the body without treatment, the more havoc it is able to play.

In the summer months and up until the first frost, it is a good idea to also add some extra Echinacea and garlic supplementation to your diet, as they are powerful natural antibiotics, along with Goldenseal Extract.

Repellants should be sprayed on clothing rather than skin to prevent absorption through the skin of toxins!

****

Here's To Your Health

by Eileen Renders N.D.   Copyright 1996

Tissue hair analysis is essential for designing a nutritional program. Hair is ideal tissue for sampling and testing. First, it can be cut easily, painlessly and can be sent to the lab without special handling requirements. Second, clinical results have shown that a properly obtained sample can give an indication of mineral status and toxic metal accumulation. A tissue mineral analysis reveals a unique metabolic world, intracellular activity, which cannot be seen through most other tests. This provides a blueprint of the biochemistry occurring during the period of hair growth and development.

A mineral imbalance can be caused by diet, stress, medications, pollution, nutritional supplements and inherited patterns.

In the seven years Renders Wellness has been in practice, we have seen juvenile diabetics who have become Calcium deficient due to their stringent watch over carbohydrate intake, along with an excess intake of diet soft drinks. We have seen individuals who are prescribed medications such as Zoloft and Prozac with excess levels of a toxic mineral such as Mercury as the culprit. Tissue Mineral Analysis can often find an iron deficiency when it has not yet shown up through a blood test. New York City's Finest Men In Blue (The N.Y. City Police) now rely on a Tissue Mineral Analysis because it is non-invasive, easy handling, and proven to be accurate!

A strong deficiency in Calcium for instance can lead to heart palpitations, insomnia, or other serious health problems. A deficiency in copper is shown to be associated with a higher risk for heart disease, and excess copper can result in Liver toxicity!

Man is composed of blood, bone, water and minerals. Each mineral, it has been determined, has an exact ratio to each of the other of the body's minerals if internal harmony, and/or optimum functioning is expected to be maintained.

Examples Of Imbalances

- Excessive intake of vitamin C can negate the beneficial effects of copper.
- Excessive vitamin D can cause a deficiency of magnesium.

- Too much iron can contribute to such symptoms as arthritis, high blood pressure, tension, headaches and dizziness.
- Taking too much calcium alone can contribute to Osteoporosis, weight gain and fatigue.
- Toxic metals can contribute to learning disabilities in children.
- Calcium loss from the body can become so advanced that severe osteoporosis can develop without any appreciable changes noted in the calcium levels in a blood test.
- Symptoms of iron deficiency can be present long before evidence can be detected in the serum.
- Excess Sodium is associated with Hypertension, but adequate amounts are required for normal health.
- Zinc is involved in the production, storage and secretion of insulin and is necessary for growth hormones.

TRACE MINERALS

By: Eileen Renders N. D.

Copyright 1999

Let's clear up a couple of facts regarding *Trace Minerals.* While they are only required in minutes amounts by the body, they are nonetheless, *essential to the proper functioning of the body.* To name a few; Cobalt (*involved with the manufacture of B-12),* lithium (*stored in minute amounts throughout the body, yet its use to man is still unknown), tungsten, strontium and etc.* These elements work in combination with various other minerals, and some of the vitamins, to stimulated (*the production of specific hormones to be released)* and/or to assist other minerals in effecting a desired response. With the above statements now made, perhaps we will have a clearer understanding of what trace minerals are, and exactly how they are used.

The second part of this article is provided in order to address a question which is frequently asked; *"What is your opinion of colloidal minerals?"* The word *c o l l o i d a l* was initially coined by a Scot chemist by the name of *T.*

Graham in 1860. The word has several meanings, however the most relevant one which pertains to colloidal means; a state of matter consisting of such a substance dispersed in a surrounding medium. All living matter contains colloidal material, and a colloid has only a negligible effect on the freezing point, boiling point, or vapor pressure of the surrounding medium. What we can deduct from that information then, is that a colloidal form of trace minerals which is available on the market today, represents a form which is easily assimilated by the human body, and can be utilized as it was intended to be. And my opinion? If you can afford it at about $29.00 a bottle, go for it! But, if you are a bit more frugal in how you spend your hard earned dollar, and would like to consider an alternative to the colloidal form, I just happen to have one for you! It is called *Kelp.* Kelp sells for about $1.99 a bottle and contains all of the trace minerals (including organic iodine), your body needs, and more. It can be used as a salt substitute(sodium chloride), and comes in a shaker bottle at your local health food store. It's iodine content is said to stimulate those with hypothyroidism, and boost the metabolism.

Caution: Excessive use of kelp can cause headaches. In such instances, back off! More is not better!

****

Vegetarians

by Eileen Renders, N.D.   Copyright 1997

Often, for personal beliefs, or because of specific health problems, many individuals choose to "Become vegetarian." While most of us have little concern for whatever motivates others, or how they arrive at transitional thresholds, as a health professional I am concerned with how a Client who becomes a vegetarian, insures his/her daily protein intake.

An example of what can and unfortunately does occur when this life-style is not thoroughly thought out, prior to implementation, can best be demonstrated by the recollection of a young woman I will refer to here as Kathy.   Kathy was a beautiful young woman in her twenties who was not feeling too good about herself, especially her weight.   Believing that she needed to lose weight, Kathy foolishly embarked upon a diet she believed would solve her problems.

For about ten days prior to being asked to see this young woman, she ate nothing at all, but a daily portion of rice. Rice without vegetables, rice without beans, or legumes. She had decided to become a Vegetarian, and lose weight. By the time I called to see this young woman she had continued what she thought was her "Diet" for ten days. Rather than lose weight however, Kathy had gained about ten pounds, was very flabby, had no energy or strength, and her eyes were listless.

What had begun to take place within her body was a breakdown of muscle in order to supply her body with the protein she was lacking. She was protein deficient, and becoming anemic. The next protein to be broken down by her body in its need to replace the protein lost, would have been her organs.

Meanwhile, Kathy did not have sufficient strength enough to lift her arms high enough to comb her beautiful long black hair, which by now had begun to lose its shine and strength and was falling out. In fact, losing her hair frightened her very much. Of course, she had no idea regarding what was going on inside her body!

All of her fear seemed to be connected with the fact that while she had recently "Become a vegetarian" to lose weight (and she was definitely not overweight), she had actually gained weight.

Upon further questioning the truth was learned, and in fact, Kathy had been eating rice as her mainstay for over a month. That knowledge, together with her symptoms, easily explained what was possibly going on. The human body has an absorption process by which nutrients in the form of glucose (from carbohydrates), amino acids (from protein), and fatty acids and glycerol (from fats) are taken up by the intestines and passed into the bloodstream to facilitate cell metabolism. All of the chemical reactions to nutrients involved in the process of metabolism of the same provides energy for new cells to be replicated, a necessary process for life. However, when we deprive the body of these essential nutrients the body's normal processes are hindered. And when the body is deprived of protein for extended periods of time (protein is necessary for building new cells and continuing life), it will soon begin to draw protein from essential muscles and organs throughout the body in the process, lean muscle is reduced to fatty tissue. And initially in the process, one may see a weight gain. Should this depravity continue, the body will take valuable protein from such organs as the heart itself.

Protein, whether it be derived from animal or plant, is necessary for the continuance of life. So before embarking into a life-style which one has little information, it is highly suggested that one learn the basics. Proper food-combination can rectify the problems, along with understanding how to supplement the needed protein the body requires.

It is worth noting here how much of these serious oversights could be eliminated when beautiful women begin to realize that their health is the most precious gift they have been given. Practicing healthier life-styles will bring the body into balance and weight will become normalized. Loving ourselves for who we are and for what we have to contribute in a positive way to the world will help us to be comfortable with who we are, and to focus our energies into being more comfortable in our own skin.

Trying to please others will leave us feeling unfulfilled, especially when we are limiting ourselves to being simply an exterior. While an interesting looking "Book jacket" may draw attention initially, most readers will agree; It is what is inside that will hold our interest and ongoing commitment to follow through..

Note: It is worth mentioning once again here that when the human body is totally deprived of protein for more than a week or ten days and longer, it will begin to break down the body's organs; Heart muscle, body muscle and etc. and consume them as a source to fulfill its immediate needs.

****

Vegetables

by Eileen Renders N.D. ~ Copyright 1998

What do you suppose are the "Healthiest" vegetables? Recent studies at the Center for Science in the Public Interest have found sweet potatoes to be the healthiest of all vegetables. The study was based on the percentage of the Recommended Daily Allowance for six months: vitamins A, C, calcium, iron, folate, and copper in each vegetable. Raw carrot was second followed by collared greens, red peppers, kale, dandelion greens, spinach and broccoli.

Tomatoes lower the risk of cancer. They neutralize uric acid found in animal products and aid in cleansing the body of toxins. While the tomato is not high in beta carotene, it does contain a high concentrate of lycopene, another type of carotene, which possibly gives the tomato its cancer protecting qualities. Peas lower cholesterol, helps to control blood sugar levels and lowers blood pressure.

Onions come from the same family as garlic, and help in the treatment of bronchitis, croup, lung infection and high blood pressure. Onions contain an acrid, volatile oil, calcium, magnesium, phosphorus, sulphur, potassium, sodium, iron, vitamins A, B and C, traces of zinc, iodine, silicon, phosphoric acids and citrate of lime.

Potatoes contain anti-cancer substances, help to lower blood pressure and assist the body in maintaining alkalinity and acidity levels within the body. Consumed raw, white potatoes contain a substance known as "Protease inhibitors" compounds known to block carcinogens. NOTE: Consumption of potatoes could be detrimental to diabetics, as they raise blood sugar levels rather quickly.

Eggplant is said to help prevent atherosclerosis, enhance immunity and prevent convulsions. And, eggplant contains a substance that inhibits the rise of blood cholesterol induced by fatty foods such as cheese. It binds up the cholesterol in the intestinal tract, so it is not absorbed into the bloodstream. It also contains substances known as acopoletin and scoparone which are said to block convulsions. NOTE: Eggplant is a nightshade vegetable, and might best be avoided by individuals who suffer from arthritis.

Chili peppers are medicinal for the lungs. They are an expectorant and decongestant, and eases chronic bronchitis and emphysema. Capsaicin, which is a substance contained in the chili pepper, is a pain killer. And chili peppers are good as a fibrinolytic stimulant, meaning they are good at preventing and dissolving blood clots.

Mushrooms lower blood cholesterol, prevent cancer, stimulate the immune system (the Shitake and Maiitake) and inactivate viruses.

Corn is brain food, good for the nervous system, and a good bone and muscle builder. It may lower cholesterol.

To cleanse the lymphatic system and to build red blood cells, eat red beets. Beets are plentiful in calcium, sodium, potassium, phosphorus, iron and magnesium. NOTE: The vitamin A, B complex and C are lost when the beet is cooked.

Horseradish is said to benefit asthma, bronchitis and lung disorders. Broccoli and Brussels sprouts lower the risk of cancer.

So, don't be a vegetable, but do eat them.

The ABC's Of Vitamins
by Eileen Renders N.D. ~ Copyright 1999

Vitamin A is a fat-soluble vitamin and was first identified as a necessary growth factor as far back as 1913. Later in 1930 it became chemically characterized by two groups of researchers, McCollum and Davis of the University of Wisconsin, and Osborne and Mendel from Yale University.

Vitamin A recently regained new recognition as a major factor involved in maintaining a healthy immune status. Carotenes, many of which are converted into vitamin A, are also a great part of that recent recognition involving vitamin A, because they have also been shown to play a role in the building of a healthy immune system.

Some of the food sources for vitamin A are liver, kidney, butter, whole milk, fortified low-fat and skim milk. Leading sources of provitamin A carotenes are in green vegetables (collards and spinach) and in yellow and orange vegetables, carrots, sweet potatoes, yams and squash. Deficiencies can arise from malabsorption due to insufficient bile acid secretion, pancreatic insufficiency, protein energy malnutrition, liver disease and several other causes.

Adult females require 800 to 4,000 International Units daily and adult males require a bit more 1,000 to 5,000 I.U.

Because the B-complex vitamins are water soluble, excesses are excreted through the body's waste system. In order for the B vitamins to properly perform their major functions throughout the body, they must all be available at the same time, because they work together as a unit, or family of workers. Supplementing them whenever a B vitamin deficiency is suspected, requires that one supplement with a B-complex vitamin.

Some of the major antagonists surrounding the B-complex vitamins (causing their supply to become depleted) are: caffeine, high amounts of refined white sugars or a diet having an over-abundance of processed foods, among other causes.

The B-complex vitamins have numerous responsibilities. Deficiencies include such symptoms as poor appetite, insomnia, high cholesterol and even depression. Supplementing with a B-complex should be included at 100 milligram dosage.

Vitamin C is essential to human health. It is a water soluble vitamin although it is a fairly stable vitamin, it is very sensitive to oxygen and can lose it's potency through exposure to light, heat or air, which can cause oxidative enzymes to activate.

While most of us know it is available in many fruits, some may not be aware that it is also found in green peppers, collard leaves, broccoli, Brussels sprouts and cabbage.

Vitamin C was long ago first recognized for it's ability to prevent Scurvy (a vitamin C deficiency) in the 1700's. Today, however, it is ever more famous for it's known ability to help aid in protecting the immune system and for assisting the body in it's attempt to remove toxins which form and accumulate throughout the body.

A good dose for a child might be about 45 milligrams daily, along with a good food source intake (especially during the cold and flu season), while for adults a couple hundred milligrams would be ideal supplemental intake, unless one is under the care and supervision of a professional.

Now that you know your ABC's, we hope that you will not forget to use them!

Weight Loss Strategies

by: Eileen Renders N. D ~ Aug., 2000

While dieting is not what we would want to promote here at Renders Wellness, we believe it is possible to stay focused on *Wellness* while taking advantage o a few healthy lifestyle habits which can stimulate weight loss. Losing weight is often the by product of healthy living, therefore it is always recommended that priority be given to maintaining optimum wellness through healthy living habits!

Remembering also to NOT have high expectations will help make your personal program a success! Often as we begin to turn body fat into muscle and to lose inches, or drop a size in clothing, our weight remains constant. Therefore, away with the scales, and don't become a victim of the scales. If you must, consider one weigh-in per week, and always at the same time of day.

Before embarking on a balanced program of nutrition and exercise, it might be a good idea to have a Mineral Hair Analysis completed. In that way, you can *see exactly where your deficiencies and imbalances are.* Severe deficiencies, or those of long standing can often lead to common disorders, and have been linked to some types of hormonal imbalances. Menopause, Adrenal exhaustion, Thyroid deficiencies and other hormonal imbalances such as poor insulin management can also contribute to weight gain, including water retention.

With the above suggested Biochemical information at hand, recommendations for adjustments can first be made which will assist in reaching one's health goals. Once that has been accomplished, and providing one does not have Heart disease, Diabetes or Digestive problems, consider adding a few of the following recommendations to your daily nutritional program;

1.   A must! ½ hour of exercise (with M..D.'S approval), walking Is safe and effective, without risk of injury. Or one hour 3 to 4 times a week. In order to lose unwanted pounds, nutritional changes will be of little benefit without *first* expending a few calories. A good way to boost the metabolism.

2.   Increase fiber (20 to 25 grams is the
suggested daily intake) through such
sources as;   Legumes (lentils, peas and
beans), whole grains, fruits, and nuts. *G
Gradually add fiber into diet in order to avoid
digestive problems; diarrhea, cramping and etc.*
Fiber is satisfying, prevents constipation and
helps to curb cravings for processed sweets.
B+ complex vitamin ~ 100 milligrams once a
day. The B-vitamins;   Niacin, Choline,
Thiamine, folic Acid and etc. are all involved
in assisting the body's effort to properly absorb
and metabolize specific nutrients, including
fats and carbohydrates, therefore they have a
positive effect upon the metabolism.

3.   Green tea extract - *Camellia sinensis) . A
study conducted by the Department of
Physiology at the University of Geneva
supported in part by the Swiss National
Research Fund, confirmed that green tea
extract promotes thermogenesis.*
Thermogenesis simply put, means the rate at
which the body burns fat. This study showed
that green tea extract's benefits far surpassed

those which might be stimulated due to any caffeine content.

4.   Conjugated linoleic acid ~ (CLA) is able to interfere with the body's storing of fat, and may also be beneficial in breaking down of fat. At the Univ. Of Wisconsin's Food Research Institute, subjects found a 20% reduction of body fat and an increase in lean body muscle after 12 weeks.

5.   Kelp ~ Belonging to the family of Seaweed, it is a good source of Iodine, a trace-mineral known for nourishing the thyroid gland. The Thyroid gland plays an important role in assisting the body maintain a healthy metabolic rate. *Note: It should be stated here that prior to embarking upon any weight loss endeavors, one should first consider that exercise is an essential part of any weight-loss plan. Therefore, it is advisable that one have a complete medical examination to determine heart health, and functioning of glands such as; Thyroid, adrenal and pancreas. For those individuals who are limited to the type of exercise they can embark upon initially, they may want to speak to their practitioner about walking or aquatic exercises.*

Wheat Germ

By: Eileen Renders N. D. ~ Copyright 1997

Recently, several clients (one associate) expressed an individual problem with taking B+Complex supplement. Though this is a rather infrequent problem, it does exist. So for those who are in need of extra B vitamins, yet cannot tolerate the usual supplements available on the market, there is an alternative.

From time to time, I have also come across those individuals who cannot metabolize the B+Complex vitamin supplements, nor the Brewer's yeast complex (which is another rich source of the B-vitamins).

For those individuals, consider wheat germ. Not only does it contain high availability of most of the B vitamins, especially thiamin, and riboflavin, but it is also plentiful in the Vitamin E. Wheat germ also contains iron.

Servings: Wheat germ contains a good portion of polyunsaturated fat, and contains approximately twenty-five percent of its calories from fat. About three tablespoons provides nine grams of protein and three grams of dietary fiber. Wheat germ rapidly turns rancid, and is nearly impossible to purchase fresh! Look for wheat germ that has been vacuum-packed and is refrigerated. Always look for a "Use by this date" label on the package. If it is impossible to find wheat germ packaged this way (or refrigerated), consider buying it toasted, as toasted wheat germ has a longer shelf life. While corn germ differs somewhat, it too can be employed in recipes such as in corn bread, fish breading, etc.

Foods containing wheat germ: Whole wheat cereals.

References

- *Adele Davis,*   *p. 21, 116*

- *American Chemical Society 1992 on Garlic*   *p. 84*

- *The Atlantic City Medical Center's HIV Consortium*   *p. 160*

- *RX ~ Prescription For Dietary Wellness By Phyllis Balch, C.N.C. & James Balch M. D. on Folic Acid*   *p. 78*

- *University of Berkley (Cancer and Exercise)*   *p. 37*

- *Dr. Stephen Barnes, Biochemist of University of Alabama on Soy*   *p. 136*

- *Dr. Johanna Budwig (Nobel Prize Nominee) On the benefits of Organic Flax Oil*   *p. 172*

- *National Cancer Institute N.I.H. Suspect List*   *p.94*

- *Stuart Richer O.D. Ph.d of North Chicago VA Medical Center on Lutein*   *p. 131*

- *T. Graham, Scot Chemist on Colloidal*   *p. 214*

- *Geriatric Medicine of The Royal Liverpool University on RLS*   *p. 113*

I

II

- *Trace Elements Inc. ~ On Biochemistry of Mineral-Hair Analysis*   *p.16, 110*
- *Dr. Watts Ph.d of Trace Elements, Inc.*   *p. 183*
- *University of Texas health and Science p.*   *168*
- *Marika Von Viczay N. D. on... The Lymphatic System*   *p. 128*
- *McCollin and Davis of The University of Wisconsin as well as Osborne and Mendel of Yale University 1930 ~ On Vitamin-A*   *p. 225*
- *University of Geneva ~ On the benefits of Green Tea*   *p. 231*
- Other Medical information regarding various disorders (including symptoms, causes, diagnosis and etc.) can be referenced in the following books;
- The Johns Hopkins Medical Handbook ~ Medical editors for John Hopkins includes Simeon Margolis., Ph.d and Hamilton Moses 111, M. D., including various contributions from dozens of physicians. Published by Random House 1992

- Fifth Edition Professional Guide To Diseases by Springhouse Publishing 1995.

****

Index

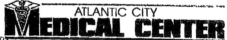

January 30, 1995

Eileen Renders, N.D.
1540 Mays Landing Rd.
Egg Harbor Township, N.J. 08234

Dear Eileen,

Thank you for agreeing to participate as a speaker for our upcoming seminar "The Menopause Issue". Please note the itinerary below and your time slot.

Subj: **Thank you for being on Voiceamerica!**
Date: 9/19/01 10:43:08 PM Eastern Daylight Time
From: skinnygirl@earthlink.net (Shannon Bishop) RD
To: erendersnd@aol.com (Eileen Renders, ND)

To: "Eileen Renders, ND"
Subject: Thank you for being on Voiceamerica!
Eileen:
What a pleasure it was to have you on the show today.
The dynamics and passion of the topic was exhilarating, to say the least!
I have had many emails come in from listeners, and people want MORE!
We have a great opportunity here, and I am more than excited.
Thanks again for your time - you were MAGNIFICENT!
I will keep in touch with future shows and possibilities...
Have a passionate & productive day!
Shannon T. Bishop, RD
Director of Nutrition & Wellness Transformations,
Inc.www.Transformations-inc.com

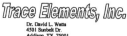

Fax! From **Trace Elements, Inc.**
Dr. David L. Watts
4501 Sunbelt Dr.
Addison, TX. 75001
Ph: 972.250.6410 Fax: 972.248.4896
E-mail: dr.watts@traceelements.com
tcilab@traceelements.com

To: Eileen Renders.   Fax: Date: 9/24/01

Re: Pages:

Dear Eileen,

I am sure that the information in this book will be of benefit to many.

Sincerely,

Dr. David L. Watts

CENTER FOR LIFESTYLE MANAGEMENT
BURDETTE TOMLIN MEMORIAL HOSPITAL

Two Stone Harbor Boulevard, Cape May Court House, NJ 08210
Telephone 609-463-2599 • FAX 609-463-2379
Dona Rè Charvet, RN BSN MA, Director

July 22, 1996

Eileen Renders
Renders Wellness
1540 Mays Landing Road
Egg Harbor Township, New Jersey 08234-8516

Dear Eileen,

On behalf of the Cancer Support Group, I would like to thank you so
much for a most enjoyable and informative presentation. Your
information was endless - we could have listened to you for hours.
You certainly raised our awareness and provoked good thought
processing regarding our eating habits.

. . .   .

AMERICAN
CANCER
SOCIETY®
New Jersey Division, Inc.
1945 ∼ 1995
Atlantic County Unit

Eileen Renders, N.D.
1540 Mays Landing Somers Point Rd.
Egg Harbor Twp. NJ 08234-8516

October 17, 1995

Dear Eileen,

Thank you, your offer to speak to our group is greatly appreciated.
You will be answering a request from the ladies. They are so
excited that you have agreed to attend our next meeting.

The cancer survivors are very interested in immunotherapy,
exercise, balance, stress reduction and healthy lifestyles. They
must be very aware of their body and their environment for a better
chance at a long and healthy life. Recurrence is a frightening
every day stress for them.

 The Children's Hospital of Philadelphia
34th Street and Civic Center Boulevard, Philadelphia, PA 19104-4399
FOUNDED 1855

Division of Oncology
(215) 590-2810 Fax (215) 590-4185

August 25, 1997

Eileen Renders, N.D.
c/o of Renders Wellness
1540 Mays Landing Road
Egg Harbor Township, NJ 08234

Re:
MR:
DOB: 10/6/89

Dear Ms. Renders.

I have had the pleasure of treating   in the Oncology
Service at Children's Hospital of Philadelphia for acute
lymphoblastic leukemia. He is currently in remission and
undergoing what we call delayed intensification chemotherapy
currently consisting of cyclophosphamide, 6-thioguanine, ara-C,
and intrathecal methotrexate. In 4 to 6 weeks he will begin the
maintenance phase of therapy consisting of monthly vincristine and
prednisone, daily 6-mercaptopurine, and weekly methotrexate by
mouth. Due to the methotrexate, folic acid in excess of RDA
should not be given.